Exercise for Seniors Strength Training Workouts

2 Books in 1

Step by Step Fully Illustrated Balance and Stretching Exercises for Fall Prevention, Improved Stability, and Posture

Robert Balazs

TABLE OF CONTENTS
BALANCE EXERCISES FOR SENIORS

STRETCHING FOR SENIORS

A Free Gift to All My Readers!

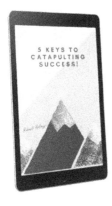 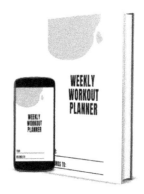

As a thank you and to help you on your fitness journey, I would love to send you a free copy of my weekly planner so that you can plan your workouts, as well as my eBook titled *5 Keys to Catapulting Success!*

To receive your complimentary copies now, please visit *www.robertbalazs.com*

Exercise Video Companionship

All of the exercises featured in this book are also available to view in video format. Not only is this book fully illustrated, but to give you the best start on your journey to better balance, I have also included a free video companion!

To get your video playlist, please visit:
https://tinyurl.com/exercisesforseniorsbundle

Balance Exercises for Seniors

Step by Step Fully Illustrated
Home Workouts for Fall Prevention,
Improved Stability, and Posture

Robert Balazs

Introduction

If you love life, don't waste time, for time is what life is made up of. –Bruce Lee

As we approach retirement, we start to look at things that we can enjoy spending our newfound freedom on. Maybe you want to travel the world or finally learn to dance. Perhaps you have always wanted to spend more quality time with your friends, children, or grandchildren. Whatever it is that you are looking forward to, you need your health on your side to be able to accomplish it.

Do you ever feel unsteady on your feet?

Have you felt like the room is moving while you are standing still?

Or have you felt lightheaded or faint?

When we have poor balance, it can be intimidating to take on social engagements, and we end up missing out on some of life's golden moments because we are too scared of the potential of sustaining injuries from falling, especially if we have already felt the effects of a developing balance disorder. Previous bad experiences can dent our confidence and we may feel like we don't want to be a burden on our families, so it would be best if we don't go to celebrations with them. The fear that feeling unstable on your feet will embarrass you or worse, cause an injury, can create a negative cycle where you do less and become more prone to accidents through lack of practice, and then more frightened.

It's important to realize, though, that you aren't alone. These kinds of problems affect many people but can also be resolved with a targeted balance training routine. One in six older Americans has a vision impairment, one in four has loss of feeling in the feet, and three in four have abnormal postural balance testing results (Dillon et al., 2010). This leads to an increased chance of falling, hip fractures, and increasing rates of heart disease and other morbidities. Additionally, balance dysfunctions are reported to physicians by 8 million adults in the U.S. (AGS Health in Aging Foundation, 2022).

The ability to balance requires the healthy functioning of several bodily systems working in coordination with each other seamlessly. It is an ability that we need to consciously learn as toddlers but that soon becomes as natural as breathing as we enter our childhood and adulthood. However, as we continue our journey into our fifties and beyond, balance starts to become something that we need to consciously put effort into again. It can stop us enjoying outings and hobbies, but it can also severely affect our daily routines, making things like shopping for groceries, moving around our homes and even showering a daunting task for some of us.

Poor balance can be the result of many things, from a central dysfunction in the body's balance centers to a lack of strength in the spine's supporting muscles. Poor core stability and recovering from injuries are also common causes. For those of us with pre-diagnosed conditions, we learn to recognize when the signs and symptoms rear their heads, but many people may not even know that a balance problem may be what is causing them to feel unwell or destabilized. The National Institute on Aging suggests that you should look out for the following common signs that could be an indication of a balance disorder:

- staggering while walking

- dizziness

- vertigo

- a feeling that you will fall

- lightheadedness

- a floating sensation

- blurred vision

- confusion

- disorientation

Anyone experiencing a sudden onset of these symptoms should consider speaking with their primary care physician for further investigation. But for many seniors, these kinds of symptoms gradually come on over time or worsen with time so slowly that you may even miss their onset all together or may not have considered associating them with one another.

As an older adult, regular physical activity is one of the most important things you can do for your health. —Centers for Disease Control and Prevention

As we age, it is inevitable that we will become somewhat less active and be less able to maintain healthy systems in our bodies. In America, only 50% of 50–64-year-old's report that they regularly exercise, with just 32% of those 65 or older taking part (Carroll, 2005). It's understandable to be wary about getting more active if you have experienced falls in the past, injuries such as rolled ankles, or have a pre-existing diagnosis of balance dysfunction. However, balance training can help to reinstate your confidence, improve your independence, and, in some cases, even reduce episodes of dizziness. Aging doesn't have to condemn you to a sedentary lifestyle or the inevitability of reduced mobility and accidents. Regular exercise for seniors can help to prevent this decline and even reverse it to a certain extent.

A healthy balance system gives you more energy and strength, and helps you move freely and confidently. –Rob Fox, YMCA fitness teacher

Research suggests that a regular commitment to balance training can bring you the following benefits:

- improved mobility

- improved posture

- increased muscle tone

- increased reaction times

- improved cognitive function

- improved core stability

- improved ability to perceive your body in relation to your surroundings

- reduced instances of falling and injuries

- increased confidence

- increased independence

- increased energy

By following along with the exercises in this book and dedicating just ten minutes a day, you can regain control of your mobility and independence, and feel fitter in the process.

I want to give you the confidence to start experiencing the joys that your hobbies, family, and friends bring you again. In this book, I show you fully illustrated exercises that will develop your key muscles for body stability and train your brain to overcome a dysfunctional ability to compensate for changes in your environment. I also cover how you adapt these exercises to suit your own health and personal goals, as well as how to make the most of equipment specially designed for improving balance.

As always, before the commencement of any sort of exercise routine or regime, please be in contact with your local healthcare provider. This is especially relevant for those with prior injuries or health issues.

Thanks for purchasing my book. After you are finished reading the book, I would really appreciate it if you could help spread the word and leave a review on Amazon so we can reach a greater audience and help them in the same way that we have hopefully helped you. To leave a review, scan the QR code below with your mobile phone and click on the book. Once you have clicked on the book, you will be able to find the button to leave a review. If you do not own a smartphone, please search for my book on Amazon and take 60 seconds to leave a review. You are amazing!

SCAN ME

About the Author

Robert Balazs was born in Canada but relocated to Scandinavia by the time he was 19. He has always had a passion for exercise, sports, and helping people.

Today, Robert is a certified personal trainer and has over a decade of experience under his belt. Over this time, he has helped hundreds of clients realize their potential and become pain-free. Helping people to achieve their health goals matters deeply to Robert, who feels it is greatly rewarding to have the privilege of witnessing people's struggles become better over time.

Robert decided to write this book when he realized that, so few seniors actually have any kind of structured exercise or training program in their daily routines. He couldn't understand how so many people were missing out on the numerous benefits of staying active and healthy into and past their 50s.

Wanting to reach and help more people is Robert's main goal in writing this book. He wants the knowledge that he has gained to help other people take control and improve their daily lives.

Chapter 1:

Balance and Its Importance

To understand what may be contributing to your balance concerns, it is important to understand what we mean when we talk about balance and why it is important for us in daily life. The word 'balance' itself refers to our ability to keep ourselves upright when sitting or standing, and our ability to properly sense the position of our bodies in relation to the ground.

When our balance is healthy, we can move around and conduct our daily tasks with little to no conscious thought. When this ability deteriorates, we consider ourselves to have poor balance. Poor balance can manifest in several ways. The symptom that most people fear is the inability to remain on their feet, which results in trips and falls. In the U.S., 3 million older people are treated for fall related injuries every year, and over 800,000 are hospitalized because of those injuries (Centers for Disease Control and Prevention, 2021).

However, trips and falls are not the only signs or symptoms of a balance issue. Other symptoms you may have started to notice include:

- unexplained dizziness

- a feeling as though you are spinning when standing still

- a feeling of floating

- feeling sick (nausea)

- a feeling as though you may pass out

- an inability to stand or sit still without assistance

These symptoms can be very frightening and may last for only an instant or up to a few days at a time. Early symptoms of balance disorders can be signs of other health conditions too. If you experience any of these symptoms for the first time without explanation or if they last more than a few days, you should contact your primary care physician for a check-up.

How Does Aging Contribute to Bad Balance?

Our bodies use several functions at once to maintain a healthy ability to balance. Due to this complexity, there are several dysfunctions that can ultimately cause or worsen balance problems. Good balance requires the normal functioning and coordination of the following bodily systems:

- **Musculoskeletal**: The physical structure of your body, the skeleton, muscles, ligaments, and tendons.

- **Nervous system**: The nerves, spinal cord, and brain.

- Proprioception: The brain's ability to understand the position of your body in space relative to your surroundings.

- **Inner ear balance center**: A collection of small organs within the ear that act as a biological spirit level for the body.

- **Vision**: The eyes, optic nerve, and vision center of the brain.

When we age, our body's natural ability to maintain itself becomes less efficient. As a result, these systems can deteriorate. Problems in each individual system can increase with age, as well as the prevalence of reported balance concerns for seniors.

Worldwide statistics show that nearly 4% of women and 3.5% of men have moderate to severe vision impairment. Those figures rise to nearly 12% and 10.5% of women and men 50 years of age or older (Elflein, 2021).

Nearly 8 million adults in the U.S. report balance problems to their physician, ⅓ of adults over 65 experience falls linked to these problems, and over half of those who are over 75 (AGS Health in Aging Foundation, 2022).

Problems with our muscles and joints can lead to poor posture and an altered stride. This is the most common cause of trips and falls. For seniors, falls are particularly concerning due to the prevalence of such an incident resulting in a fractured hip. More than 300,000 older people are hospitalized each year due to hip fractures (Centers for Disease Control and Prevention, 2021).

What are the Benefits of Exercise to Combat This?

Staying active is a key component to improving balance and preventing falls. Our sedentary lifestyles go against the natural evolution of our bodies and can lead to weakened muscles, poor posture, and loss of coordination.

Studies show that six weeks or more of balance training exercises can reduce the occurrence of lower limb injuries, such as ankle or knee sprains, as well as speed up the healing process after receiving a sprain (McKeon et al., 2008). However, it is recommended to train your balance for at least 11–12 weeks to get the maximum benefit from your exercise. These kinds of studies remind us of the importance of an effective ability to balance and show how the lower limbs in particular can be a crucial part of improving your balance. Muscles that stabilize your ankles and knees, along with core stability muscles in your abdomen and back, must function in perfect coordination to maintain your position when standing or walking. When any of these are working out of sync with the others, the instance of falls increases.

Exercising to improve your balance has several health benefits, including:

- Helping to reduce the effects of aging on balance.

- Improving coordination to better recover from slips and prevent falls.

- Improved posture and reduced posture related pain.

- Improves your walking technique to better handle uneven surfaces, such as walking on gravel or uphill.

- Increasing the strength of muscles.

- Reducing the likelihood of lower limb injuries.

- Improving confidence in standing or walking.

Other Things That Can Help Prevent Falls

Though balance training exercises are important in helping you to become more confident and prevent falling, there are other ways you can improve your safety alongside your exercise program. As we discussed, balance requires the coordination of many functions in your body to work efficiently. We can counter the effects of dysfunction in these areas with proper medical attention from your primary care physician or ophthalmologist. For example, having your eyesight and hearing regularly tested and properly using any glasses or hearing aids provided will help you to have the best possible understanding of your environment while you are moving around it.

Sometimes our balance is affected by drugs. If you are at risk of falling, you should limit the amount of alcohol that you drink, as it can negatively affect your coordination. Besides recreational activities, prescription medication can sometimes have side effects that include dizziness or confusion. It is important that you read all the documentation given to you with your medication to be aware of any such side effects. If a medication is making you feel overly dizzy or sleepy, you should consult your physician to see if they can provide a counter measure, or alternative.

If you require the help of a walking aid, don't be embarrassed to use it, but do be sure that you are aware of the correct way in which it should be used. If you do require the help of a walking aid, you aren't alone, and you certainly aren't any less of a person because of it. 25% of older Americans use either a cane, walker, wheelchair, or scooter (Huffman, 2015).

Health conditions such as diabetes, heart disease, and high or low blood pressure can contribute to falls, so it is important to understand your condition and how it affects you in daily life if you have any additional health needs. It is important to be sure that you stand slowly to prevent a fall in your blood pressure and dizziness. Be sure to get enough sleep too, as feeling sleepy can also contribute to poor balance.

Now that we have covered your health and body, I want to give you some tips on making sure that your environment is as safe as possible and making sure you are properly equipped to handle outside environments too. Keeping your home's walkways clear of clutter is a simple but effective way to make it easier to get around your home safely. If you have any pets, be sure to keep a lookout for them when you are walking through your home and let them go ahead of you where possible to reduce the risk of them causing you to trip.

Your choice of footwear is important both in the home and when you are out and about doing errands. Be sure to avoid walking around the house in socks alone; a good pair of shoes is best. If you absolutely can't live without a cozy pair of slippers, get yourself a pair with a rubber non-slip sole and a style that covers your whole foot. Avoid backless slippers. When choosing your shoes, look for styles that are low-heeled, non-skid, and have a sole that is thick enough to protect you from objects that may be on the floor, but thin enough so that you can still feel the surface beneath your feet. Avoid wearing platform shoes. They may look safe as they don't hold your feet in a high-heel position, but the large sole will stop you from being able to properly sense the position of your feet in relation to the floor.

Whenever you go somewhere new that you are not familiar with, take your time to make your way around. Be extra vigilant when it is icy out or the floor is wet. Both conditions can make the ground very slippery and dangerous. Save some sand and salt so that you can spread it near your front and back doors, or along any paths in your garden to improve the way your shoes will grip the surface.

Chapter 2:

Testing Your Balance

What to Expect From This Book

Who is This Book For?

I wrote this book with the intention of spreading knowledge of how to improve balance and reduce the risk of falling for seniors or anyone who is experiencing a reduced ability to balance following an injury or illness. This book is for all those who want to get ahead with their balance skills, prevent falls from occurring, and increase confidence in their mobility. It can also be a great source of information for anyone who has a loved one with any of the conditions listed above who they want to be able to help.

What Types of Exercises are in This Book?

This book contains exercises aimed at strengthening your muscles and training your balance centers to improve your posture and, in turn, increase your stability while sitting or standing. The exercises are grouped into the following three types:

- Sitting: A great place to start if you fear losing your balance while standing, so that you can still feel safe while developing your posture.

- Standing: Practicing movements that combine to create your walking style and improve your strength.

- Vestibular: Carefully chosen to retrain your balance centers, improving your brain's ability to comprehend how your body relates to the world around you.

All the exercises I have included in this book can be scaled up to really push your ability to the next level, once you have familiarized yourself with the base routines. Similarly, if you have already experienced falls, sustained injuries, or suffered illnesses such as a stroke, which is currently limiting your ability to perform these exercises, can be scaled down so that you can still start to retrain your balance safely.

How to Use This Book?

Before you start any new exercise routine or training plan, you should always consult your primary care physician or other health professional to ensure that it is safe and correct for your individual health situation.

The exercises in this book are intended to be done daily. Choose ten of the exercises each day and keep rotating through them, both to ensure that you target every area of improvement in your balance and to keep things interesting. If you enjoy your routine, you will be more likely to stick to it. Once you feel like you are confident with each exercise, move onto the advanced exercises and consider adding in balance tools to take your training up a notch.

When Should You Train Your Balance?

The key to seeing good results is consistency. Building a routine that you can stick to every day will help you get the most out of your balance training. It is important that you check your diary or planner to select a time of day that you can stick to regularly. Please visit my webpage now to get your free copy of my weekly planner to help you start planning your new routine today (*www.robertbalazs.com*).

Practicing your exercise routine first thing in the morning after you wake up can help to boost your mood and prepare you for the day ahead. Alternatively, planning your routine before bedtime can relieve any tension that you may have built up during the day, helping you relax and get a better night's sleep. Ultimately, you will know which times feel right for you. Don't be afraid to change your time if you feel it isn't right. It is better to change your routine so that you are comfortable and will stick with it, than to feel uncomfortable while you train and ultimately feel like giving up.

Testing Your Balance

Below are four exercises that you can use to test your current ability to balance. They can be used as a tool to measure the improvement in your balance as you progress on your exercise journey. For safety reasons, it is important that you conduct these exercises with a sturdy chair nearby, so that you can grab onto it if you feel yourself starting to lose your balance or feel lightheaded.

How to use these exercises to measure your improvement:

1. Perform each exercise, holding the position for as long as you can before you are forced to correct your posture by moving a foot or arm out to save your balance.

2. Use a stopwatch or other timer to time the length of your hold.

3. Record the times that you get for each exercise.

4. Repeat the exercises once a week and compare your times to the previous week, so that you can see your improvement.

Feet Together Eyes Closed

1. Stand straight with your feet together.

2. Keep your arms by your sides and close your eyes.

3. Hold this position for as long as possible and record the length of time that you can stay here without needing to step aside to rebalance or grab onto a chair or counter.

You will feel your body swaying when your eyes are closed. This is normal, but if you feel yourself starting to fall or feel dizzy, then open your eyes and stop. You may want to take a seat until you feel better.

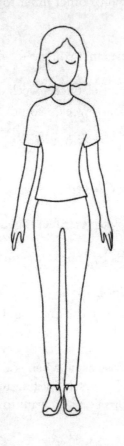

Single Leg Hold

1. Stand straight with your feet together.

2. Keep your arms by your sides.

3. Bend one leg 90 degrees at the knee.

4. Hold this position for as long as possible and record the length of time you can stay here without needing to put your foot back on the floor.

5. For an accurate representation of your balance repeat this with your other leg and record that time too.

Be sure to keep your arms by your sides, avoid the temptation to hold your raised leg with your hand. However, if you feel any pain in your knees or ankles, you should stop this test until you have worked on strengthening your legs.

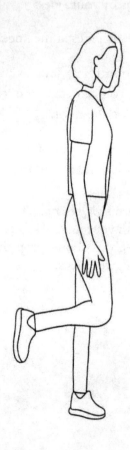

Tandem Stance

1. Stand straight with your feet together.

2. Keep your arms by your sides.

3. Place your right foot in front of your left, bringing your foot to the center line and touching the heel of the right foot to the toes of the left foot.

4. Hold this position for as long as possible and record the length of time you can stay here without needing to step out and regain your balance.

5. For an accurate representation of your balance, repeat this with your left foot in front of your right foot and record that time too.

Be sure to keep your feet on the center line in front of one another, avoiding letting your toes point outwards or stepping too far forward.

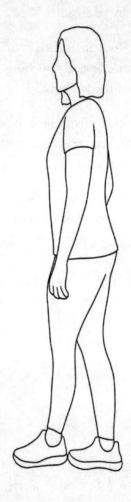

Chapter 3:

Getting Started

Preparing for Success

Equipment Needed

Athletic clothing: Choose clothing that is breathable but not too loose. Cotton or specialist athletic clothes with breathable materials are a good choice. You will want to choose items that allow you to move freely while exercising, but avoid clothing that is too long in the arms or legs.

Appropriate footwear: Either exercise in bare feet or choose a pair of shoes with a flat sole that will support the arch of your foot and ankles. Your footwear should be properly laced or otherwise fastened to prevent it slipping off.

Water bottle: Sufficient hydration is critical to a safe and effective workout. Be sure to keep a water bottle nearby and take regular sips between exercises. You will lose water through your sweat, so drinking enough to replace this will be important.

Chair: You will need to have a sturdy chair handy when exercising. Be sure to choose a chair that is free from any damage and that connects soundly to the floor through all four legs. Look for a chair with a solid seat. A dining chair is a good example. Avoid using a sofa, as this can lead to slouching and a reduced ability to perform the full movement of the exercise.

Towel: Different people will experience different amounts of sweating while they exercise. However much you sweat, it is a good idea to keep a towel handy so that you can wipe it away and stay comfortable.

Music: If you prefer to exercise with music playing, choose some that will keep you motivated or relaxed, to your taste. Whichever music you choose, be sure to prepare it before you start. Getting distracted by choosing or skipping songs mid-exercise can lower your motivation to continue.

What Should Your Exercise Schedule Look Like?

I always recommend that you start out slowly and increase your exercise as you progress along your fitness journey. Balance training can be taxing, so it's best to ease into your full routine in stages. Start with two to three sessions per week. You can add in another session each week until you reach a full daily routine. Remember that exercise should be enjoyable, if you feel pain ease back and take a rest, check that you are correctly doing your technique so that you don't overexert yourself. There is no shame in sticking to just a few sessions a week for as long as you feel you need to, especially if you are already diagnosed with a balance disability (dysfunction) or have an injury.

Where and How to Set Up

The exercises in this book can be performed anywhere, but there are some things you need to consider before getting started. Choose a space to exercise in that has a comfortable temperature and sufficient heating or air conditioning depending on the season.

If you feel uncomfortable exercising in front of people, opt for an exercise space that has some privacy.

I recommend avoiding hard flooring such as concrete or tile, but if you can't avoid this, it is fine to counteract this by using an exercise mat or blanket. If you need to use blankets, be sure not to choose thick or layered blankets such as duvets, as they can shift underfoot and negatively affect your balance.

Be sure to clear your exercise space of any clutter before you start. You may also want to ensure that any pets are placed in another room to avoid potential accidents from them getting underfoot.

Before you start, take a moment to get into the correct frame of mind. Build some anticipation for the things you will soon be able to do independently again. Go into your new routine with a winning mindset, and don't forget your water bottle.

The Importance of Breathing

A common mistake that people make while exercising is holding their breath through the movements. This reduces the efficiency of your exercise in several ways. Firstly, it makes you feel out of breath more quickly, but it also limits the amount of movement available for you to use during your exercise around your chest and back. Holding your breath can tighten your muscles and result in poor function as it lowers the amount of oxygen available for them to utilize in movement.

For the exercises I have chosen for you, I recommend consistent and controlled breathing. Keep a regular pace, breathing in through your nose and out through your mouth. If you ever notice yourself holding your breath, stop and take a deep breath in, let it out in a sigh, do this three times, and then restart your exercise. This is intended to refocus you on your breathing. If this is unsuccessful and you find you return to holding your breath, it could be a sign that you are finding exercise too strenuous, and you should consider adapting it to make it easier for yourself until you are able to increase the intensity again.

Warming Up

Warming up before you exercise is a keyway to improve the results of your exercise and reduce the likelihood of injury by preparing your body for the work it is about to do. It gets your blood pumping by increasing your heart rate and starts to transport more oxygen to your muscles so that they are ready to perform for you. It's also a good way of getting you into the right mindset for your exercise routine by triggering the thought that it's time to work out now.

I have included three warm-ups for you that are ideal to prepare your body for balance training. However, if you find them too difficult, they can be substituted for general warm-up techniques such as walking, running, or spinning. If you choose to substitute for any of these more conventional techniques, I recommend that you do them for at least five minutes to sufficiently raise your heart rate and body temperature.

For the warm-ups below, perform each one for 40 seconds—take a 20-second break, and then repeat. Take another break and then move onto the next warm-up. If you choose to incorporate the full routine, it will take you six minutes to complete.

Seated Hip Circles

Areas Targeted: Hips, abdomen, and back muscles; visual input, and proprioception—particularly the balance structures in the ear.

1. Sit in your chair with your feet hip width apart.

2. Place your hands on your hips with your elbows bent out to your sides.

3. Lean to your left and then forwards, rotating your torso above your hips.

4. Move your torso across to the right and back up to a tall, seated position.

5. Repeat the circle for 20 seconds, then switch directions.

6. Lean to your right and then forwards, rotating your torso above your hips.

7. Move your torso across to the left and back up to a tall, seated position.

8. Repeat the circle for 20 seconds.

9. Take a 20-second break and then repeat.

The goal is to draw a circle in the air with your shoulders so that it creates a circular motion around your hips. Try to make your circles as deep as possible but keep your bottom fully on the seat. Avoid curling or arching your back as far as possible. You want to aim to generate the movement from your hips and not your spine. If you feel unsteady during this exercise, you can place your hands on the sides of the chair for support but be sure not to drive the circles from your shoulders if you do this.

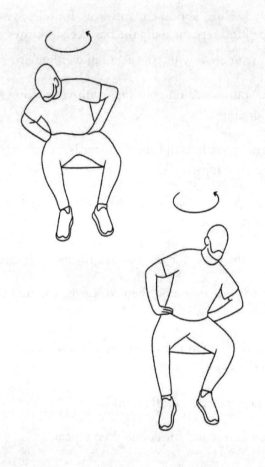

Seated Hip Leans

Areas Targeted: Hips, abdomen, neck, and back muscles, visual input and proprioception—particularly the balance structures in the ear.

1. Sit in a chair with your feet hip width apart.

2. Place your hands on your hips with your elbows bent out to your sides.

3. Lean forwards bending at the hip as far as you comfortably can.

4. Slowly sit up straight.

5. Repeat leaning forwards and back for 40 seconds.

6. Take a 20-second break and then repeat.

The aim of this warm-up is to bend at the hip, avoiding curling your back as you move. To keep the movement controlled throughout, you may want to pause briefly at your furthest point forward and when you sit back upright, this will help you to avoid getting into a swinging motion that is relying on momentum rather than poise. If you find this too difficult, you can support yourself by placing your hands on either side of the chair. If you choose to do this, avoid pushing yourself forward with your arms.

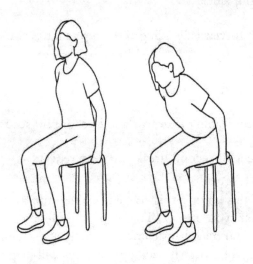

Seated Marches

Areas Targeted: Hips, abdomen, thigh muscles, and proprioception.

1. Sit in a chair with your feet hip width apart.

2. Place your arms down by your sides.

3. Lift your left leg, keeping your knee bent.

4. Lower your left leg, then lift your right leg, keeping your knee bent.

5. Lower your right leg.

6. Repeat this action, alternating from one leg to the other for 40 seconds.

7. Take a 20-second break and then repeat.

Lift your knees as high as you comfortably can but be sure not to allow your legs to fall out to the sides as you do. You will want to alternate as quickly as you can without overexerting yourself, as this exercise is particularly good for raising your heart rate. As with the other warm-ups, if you find this too difficult, you can support yourself by holding either side of the chair. Be sure not to hold your arms rigidly if you do this, as it may encourage you to hold your breath, which you need to avoid doing.

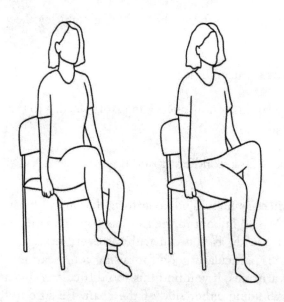

Chapter 4:

Seated Exercises

Seated Arm Lifts

Areas Targeted: Shoulder, upper arm, back, abdomen muscles, and proprioception.

1. Sit upright in a chair with your feet hip-width apart.

2. Spread your knees slightly to allow your hands to touch the flat section of the seat in front of you.

3. Cup your right hand with your left hand and, with both hands together slowly raise your arms in front of you and then up over your head.

4. Slowly lower your arms.

5. Then raise them again. This time, keep them pointing forward but move slightly out to the side. Ending with your hands in the air above your head approximately in line with your right shoulder so that your back is curved slightly to the right.

6. Slowly lower your arms and then repeat, aiming to end with your arms above your head approximately in line with your left shoulder and your back slightly curved to the left.

7. Repeat this set of three times for a total of eight.

If you are struggling when you first start, you can make this exercise easier by only raising your arms halfway. If necessary, you can aim to only reach the height of your shoulders. Try to avoid twisting your torso. The aim is to keep your shoulders facing forwards as you lift your arms.

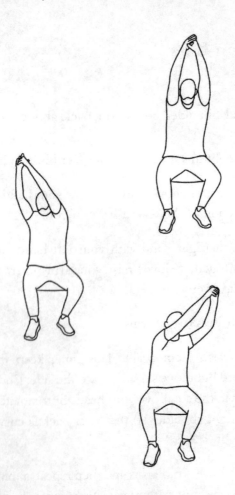

Cup Toe Tap

Areas Targeted: Hips, abdomen, thigh muscles, and proprioception.

1. Place a cup on the floor in front of you, in line with the middle of your chair.

2. Sit upright in your chair and tuck your heels in towards the front legs of the chair.

3. Lift your right leg and move it into the center tapping your toes on top of the cup.

4. Return your right leg back to the ground in front of the chair leg.

5. Lift your left leg and move into the center tapping your toes on top of the cup.

6. Return your left leg to the ground in front of the chair leg.

7. Alternate each leg until you have completed eight taps on each side.

Try to avoid moving your legs too far away from your cup or out to the side whenever you return your foot to the ground. Also, be sure that your cup is centered in front of you. You can make this exercise easier or more difficult by lowering or raising the height of the cup that you choose.

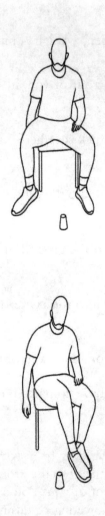
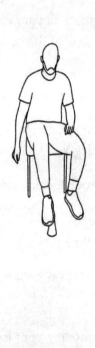

Seated Arm and Leg Lifts

Areas Targeted: Hips, thighs, abdomen, back, shoulder muscles, coordination, and proprioception.

1. Sit in your chair with your feet hip width apart.

2. Raise your right arm and right leg at the same time, keep your arm straight and your leg bent at the knee at 90 degrees.

3. Lower your right arm and right leg at the same time, then swap sides.

4. Raise your left arm and left leg at the same time, keep your arm straight and your leg bent at the knee at 90 degrees.

5. Lower your left arm and left leg.

6. Continue alternating each side of your body until you have completed eight lifts on each side.

If you find it too difficult to alternate from side to side, you can make this exercise a little easier by completing eight repetitions on one side first and then switching to do eight repetitions on the other. Aim to lift your arm right up above your head and bring your knee as close to your chest as you can manage. Avoid allowing your torso to bend to the side or allowing your body to tip over to the side that you are currently raising in the air.

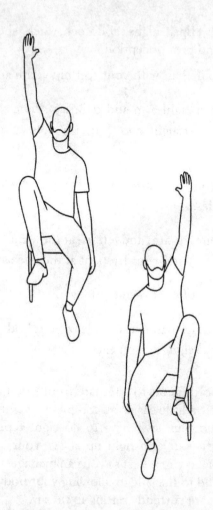

Torso Rotation Leg Openers

Areas Targeted: Hips, abdomen, back, thigh, buttocks muscles, and proprioception.

1. Sit upright in your chair with your feet hip apart.

2. Slide your left leg out to the side of the chair until your legs are at right angles to one another at the hip.

3. Then twist your torso to the right so that you are feeling a light stretch around your left hip area.

4. Twist your torso back to the center then return your left leg to its resting position in front of you.

5. Slide your right leg out to the side of the chair until your legs are at right angles to one another at the hip.

6. Then twist your torso to the left so that you are feeling a light stretch around the right hip area.

7. Twist your torso back to the center and then return your right leg to its resting position in front of you.

8. Continue alternating from side to side until you have completed eight twists in either direction.

Aim to twist your torso so that you can look over the back of the chair. It is fine if you cannot twist this far when you are first starting out. If you are finding this exercise difficult, you can support your upper torso by placing your arms on your extended knee and the back of the chair for support. However, avoid using your arms to pull your body into a twist. The movement should come from your hips and spine only. You may experience pain in your inner hip, especially if you stand or sit still for long periods of time. If this is the case, you can reduce the intensity by either reducing the degree of your torso rotation or by sliding your leg a shorter distance, thus reducing the angle between your legs.

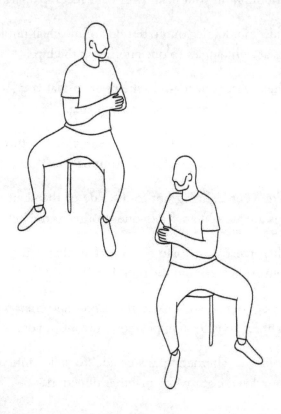

Forward Reach to the Ankle Tap

Areas Targeted: Hips, abdomen, back, shoulders, buttocks, thighs, and calf muscles; coordination; visual input; and proprioception—particularly the balance structures in the ear.

1. Sit upright in your chair with your feet hip width apart.

2. Slide your right foot forwards, straightening your leg and keeping the sole of your foot flat on the floor.

3. With your left arm, reach forward and over your center to touch the inside of your right ankle.

4. Return to an upright position then slide your right foot back towards the chair.

5. Slide your left foot forwards, straightening your leg and keeping the sole of your foot flat on the floor.

6. With your right arm, reach forward and over your center to touch the inside of your left ankle.

7. Return to an upright position then slide your left foot back towards the chair.

8. Continue alternating from side to side until you have completed eight ankle taps on each side.

You may experience some pain at the back of your knee, in your calves, or hamstrings if you are used to standing still a lot. To reduce this, you can reduce the distance that you slide your feet away from the chair and keep your knees slightly bent. And when you lean forward, be sure that most of the movement is happening at your hips and try to avoid curling your spine over your knee.

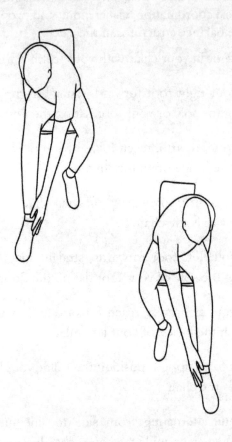

Chapter 5:

Standing Exercises

Side Leg Raise

Areas Targeted: Hips, abdomen, back, buttocks, outer thigh muscles, coordination, visual input, and proprioception.

1. Stand with your feet hip width apart.

2. Place your hands on your waist with a bend at your elbows.

3. Lift your right leg out to the side keeping your knee straight.

4. Then lower your right leg back to the floor.

5. Lift your left leg out to the side keeping your knee straight.

6. Then lower your left leg back to the floor.

7. Continue alternating sides until you have completed eight raises with each leg.

Your torso will naturally lean a little to the opposite side of the leg that you are raising. However, be sure not to allow yourself to bend sideways at the waist. Also, avoid allowing your torso to lean so far that you feel you will topple over. If you are finding this difficult, you can perform this exercise standing in front of a kitchen counter, which you can hold for support.

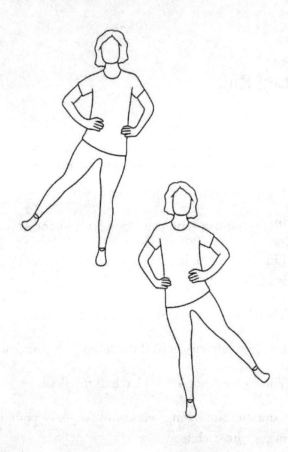

Forward Heel Taps

Areas Targeted: Hips, ankles, knees, back muscles, coordination, visual input, and proprioception.

1. Stand with your feet hip width apart and your arms at your sides.

2. Step forwards with your right foot allowing only the heel to make contact with the floor.

3. Return your right foot to your original hip width stance.

4. Then step forward with your left foot allowing only the heel to make contact with the floor.

5. Return your left foot to your original hip width stance.

6. Continue alternating feet until you have completed eight heel taps on each side.

Aim to keep your ankle bent so that your toes point slightly upwards when you tap your heel on the floor. However, the more that you bend your ankle upwards, the more difficult this exercise will become. If you are finding this difficult, you can moderate the exercise by taking smaller steps or, if need be, by touching your heel to the opposite toes only and then returning to your hip width stance. And you can also perform this exercise standing next to a wall facing sideways onto it so that when you step forward you do so parallel to the wall and can support yourself by placing your hand against the wall.

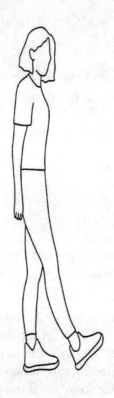

Side Toe Taps

Areas Targeted: Hips, knees, ankles, abdomen, back, buttock muscles, coordination, visual input, and proprioception.

1. Stand with your feet hip width apart and your hands at your sides.

2. Step out to the side using your right foot.

3. Allow your left knee to bend so that your right step can be larger, tap your right toes to the floor at your side.

4. Bring your right foot back into your hip width stance.

5. Then step out to the side using your left foot allowing your right knee to bend so the step can be larger.

6. Bring your left foot back into your hip width stance.

7. Continue alternating sides until you have completed eight toe taps on each side.

Remember that the larger you make your steps, the lower you will need to dip by bending your opposite knee and the more difficult this exercise will become. In the beginning, if you are finding this exercise too difficult, you can stand in front of a kitchen counter and hold onto it for support. While doing this exercise, remember to keep your back straight and do not allow yourself to bend over towards either side.

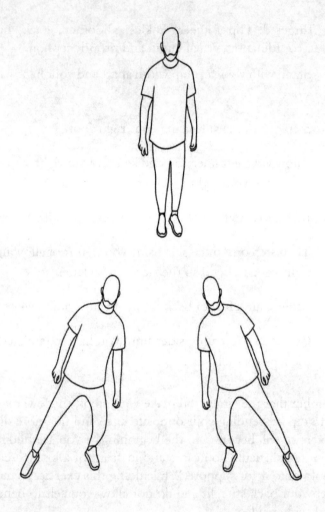

Heel Raise

Areas Targeted: Ankles, knees, buttocks, calf muscles, and proprioception.

1. Stand with your feet hip width apart behind the back of a chair.

2. Hold the back of your chair with both hands for support.

3. Raise both heels off the floor at the same time until you are on your tiptoes.

4. Then lower your heels back to the ground.

5. Repeat this process 10 times.

If you are finding this exercise difficult, you can reduce the height that you raise your heel from the ground. For safety reasons, I recommend a chair be used for this exercise. Aim to keep your ankles, knees, and hips in a straight line up from the floor. By this, I mean avoid allowing your joints to bow out to the sides or into the middle whilst you raise your heels.

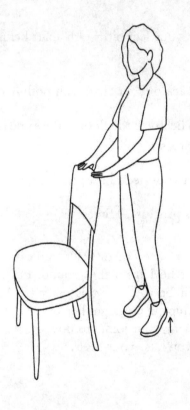

Toe Raise

Areas Targeted: Ankles, knees, buttocks, calf muscles, and proprioception.

1. Stand with your feet hip width apart behind the back of a chair.

2. Hold the back of the chair with both hands for support.

3. Raise the balls of your feet on both sides at the same time so that you are lifting your toes towards the ceiling.

4. Lower your toes back to the floor.

5. Repeat this process 10 times.

You may find that you bend slightly at the hip to allow yourself to continue holding the back of the chair. A small bend is fine, but avoid a tendency to squat downwards. If you are finding this exercise difficult, remember that the higher you lift the toes, the harder it will become. Therefore, you can reduce the intensity when you first begin by doing smaller sized toe raises.

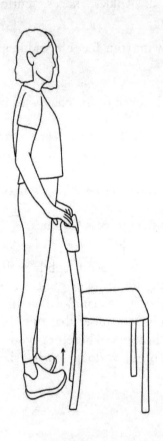

Lean Forward

Areas Targeted: Hips, abdomen, back, and shoulder muscles; coordination; visual input; and proprioception—particularly the balance structures in the ear.

1. Stand with your feet hip-width apart.

2. Touch the inside edges of your wrists together with your fingers pointing forwards and raise your arms out in front of you until they are level with your shoulders.

3. Lean your torso forward until your shoulders cross an imaginary line made by the front of your toes.

4. Stand back upright and pause.

5. Then lean forwards again and repeat the lean eight times.

The further forwards that you lean the more off center your weight will be balanced and the more difficult the exercise will become. Remember that your hips might bend slightly backwards while you do this. A small bend is fine, but avoid allowing your hips to take over the motion. You want to reach forward and not squat backwards. If you are finding this exercise too difficult, you can adapt it by completing the leans without your arms stretched in front of you.

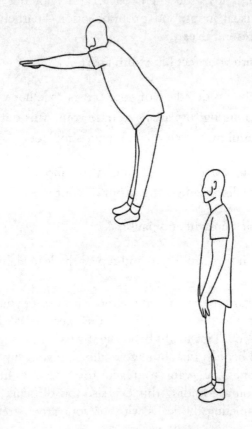

Side Lean

Areas Targeted: Hips, abdomen, back, shoulders, and muscles at the sides of the chest; coordination; visual input; and proprioception—particularly the balance structures in the ear.

1. With your feet hip width apart and your arms at your sides.

2. Raise your left arm out to your left side until it is parallel to the floor.

3. Then lean your torso towards your left.

4. Stand back upright then lower your arm.

5. Switch sides to raise your right arm until it is parallel with the floor.

6. Lean your torso towards the right.

7. Stand back upright then lower your arm.

8. Continue alternating sides until you have completed eight leans on each side.

Remember that when you lean to the side, you should be bending your spine, allowing your hips to bend out backwards. If you are finding this exercise too difficult, you can moderate the complexity by completing the side lean without your arms stretched out to the side.

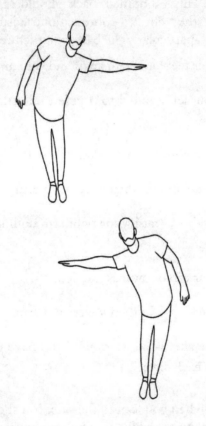

Tandem "Side to Side"

Areas Targeted: Ankles, hips, abdomen, back, neck muscles, visual input, and proprioception.

1. Stand with your feet one in front of the other, touching the heel of your front foot to the toes of your back foot. It doesn't matter which foot is in front you can choose whichever is most comfortable.

2. Keep your arms by your side and turn your head to face the left until you are looking over your left shoulder.

3. Turn your head back to the center and then turn your head to the right until you are looking over your right shoulder.

4. Turn your head back to the center so that you are facing forwards.

5. Keep alternating the side that you look at until you have turned each way eight times.

Try to avoid allowing your torso to twist. The aim of this exercise is to turn your head so that you are looking away from the direction that your body is pointing. If you are finding this exercise difficult, you can begin by standing sideways parallel to a wall and supporting yourself with one hand on the wall. If you experience vertigo, you might find this exercise particularly difficult. However, if you do not experience any dizziness, it is fine for you to still practice this movement.

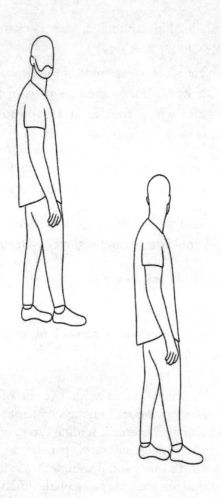

Rock the Boat

Areas Targeted: Ankles, knees, hips, abdomen, and back muscles; coordination; visual input and proprioception—particularly the balance structures in the ear.

1. Stand with your feet shoulder width apart.

2. Keeping your hands at your sides, lift your left foot off the ground keeping your knee straight and allowing your weight to rock over onto your right leg.

3. Rock back onto your left leg as you return your foot to the floor, then lift your right leg allowing your weight to transfer to your left.

4. Continue alternating sides until you have completed eight rocks in each direction.

The aim of this exercise is that you keep your back straight and do not bend to lean to the side. Rather, what you are looking for is a stiff looking movement that resembles that of a rocking chair, the exception being that this movement is side to side rather than backwards and forwards. When you lift your leg, raise it as far as you can from the ground without losing your balance. If you are finding this exercise difficult, you can adapt it by reducing the height to which you lift your legs.

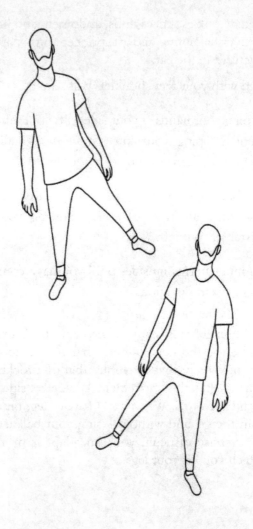

A Giant Backwards Step

Areas Targeted: Ankles, knees, hips, abdomen, back, thigh, and calf muscles; coordination; visual input; and proprioception—particularly the balance structures in the ear.

1. Stand with your feet hip width apart.

2. Place your hands on your waist with your elbows bent.

3. Step backwards on your left foot. Make the step as large as possible, bending the right knee to accommodate the large distance of the backward step.

4. Return your left foot to your resting hip-width position.

5. Step backwards onto your right foot, bending your left knee to allow you to make as large a step as possible.

6. Return your right foot to your resting hip-width position.

7. Continue alternating each side until you have completed eight giant steps with each leg.

Aim to keep the front leg pointing forwards and avoid allowing your knee to tip outwards to the side. Be sure to securely plant the ball of your back foot on the ground as you take your giant backward step. You don't want to touch the top of your foot to the floor, as this may over stretch your ankle. If you are finding this exercise difficult, you can reduce the intensity by taking smaller steps. However, this will also reduce the effectiveness, so I recommend only doing this for a few sessions and gradually increasing the size of your steps as you go along.

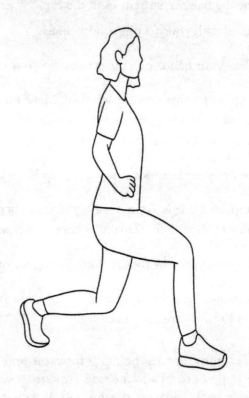

Chapter 6:

Walking Exercises

Tightrope Walk

Areas Targeted: Ankles, knees, hips, abdomen, and back muscles; visual input; coordination and proprioception.

1. Stand straight with your arms at your sides.

2. Move your left foot in front of your right foot, touching your left heel to your right toes, forms a straight line forward with both feet.

3. Next, move your right foot to step in front of your left. Touch your right heel to your left toes.

4. Continue stepping forward, one foot in front of the other until you have achieved 20 steps.

The aim is to walk in as straight a line as possible while keeping your balance. Imagine that you are walking on a tightrope or that you have a line painted on the floor that you must follow, like a sobriety test. You can look at your feet to help you get the placement correct, but over time, the aim would be to be able to walk 20 steps with your head held high, looking forward. If you find this exercise particularly difficult, you can perform it by walking alongside your kitchen counters so that you have a surface to hold onto if you are feeling unsteady.

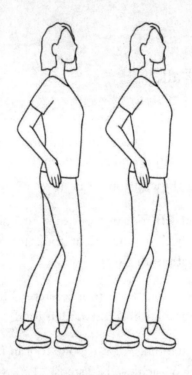

High Knee Marches

Areas Targeted: Ankles, knees, hips, thighs, buttocks, abdomen, and back muscles, visual input, and proprioception.

1. Stand straight with your arms at your sides.

2. Raise your left leg in the air, bending at least 90 degrees at both the hip and knee.

3. Place your left foot down in front of you.

4. Transfer your weight to your left leg and swap sides.

5. Raise your right leg in the air, bending at least 90 degrees at both the hip and knee.

6. Place your right foot down in front of you.

7. Walk forwards raising your knees as high as you can before setting your feet down onto the floor in front of you with each step.

8. Continue repeating this exaggerated step, alternating the leg that you step forward with until you have completed 20 steps.

The aim of this exercise is to practice balancing for a longer time on one leg while still moving forward. It will develop your ability to confidently make large strides when walking on slopes, upstairs, or anywhere else that there is uneven ground. Try to raise your knees as high as you can and keep looking ahead as you march. There is no need to swing your arms, but if you find it helpful in the beginning, you can do so. Just remember that you don't want the momentum of your arms to pull you along. As with the tightrope walk, if you are finding this difficult, it is okay to perform alongside the line of your kitchen counters for security.

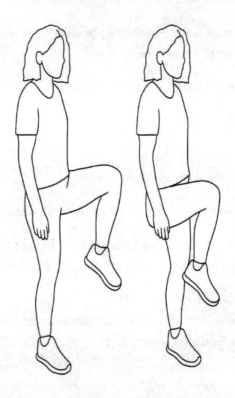

Crossovers

Areas Targeted: ankles, knees, hips, thighs, buttocks, abdomen, and back muscles; visual input; coordination; and proprioception.

1. Stand straight with your feet hip-width apart.

2. Cross your left leg in front of your right leg, stepping your foot out to your right side.

3. Then follow with your right leg to the right, undoing the crossing of your legs as you do so.

4. Step your left leg to the right again this time crossing your leg behind your right leg.

5. Undo the cross of your legs once more by stepping your right leg out to the right side.

6. Then reverse your direction of travel. Start by crossing your right leg in front of your left leg and out to your left side.

7. Uncross your legs by stepping your left leg out to the left.

8. Cross your legs again by passing the right leg behind your left leg to step to the left.

9. Uncross your legs by stepping your left leg out to the left side.

10. Repeat this pattern of crossing and uncrossing your legs until you have achieved the full motion four times in each direction, creating eight crossovers with one leg in front and eight crossovers with one leg behind.

This exercise is very similar to a dance move that is sometimes known as the 'grapevine.' Its intention is for you to practice switching your weight from one leg to the other in more than one plane of movement, without necessarily traveling forward. This will help you get used to keeping stable when walking on uneven surfaces, as well as practice training your brain to recognize where your feet are in the space around you. If you are finding this exercise difficult, you can perform it in front of a wall so that you can reach out to support yourself if needed. Try to avoid looking down at your feet, as this can disorientate you since you're making an unusual pattern of steps.

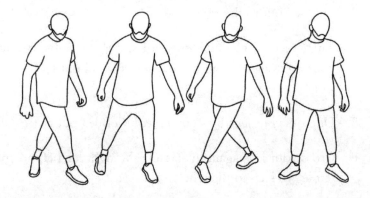

Sidesteps

Areas Targeted: Ankles, knees, hips, thighs, and buttock muscles; visual input; and proprioception.

1. Stand with your feet hip-width apart.

2. Move your left leg out to the side, creating a wide sidestep, notice that your body will become closer to the ground to account for the new wider stance.

3. Bring your right leg to meet your left leg so that you are standing upright with your feet hip-width apart again.

4. Repeat the step to the left re-making a wide stance and then closing the stance by bringing your right foot in to meet your left foot.

5. Now switch directions. Move your right leg out to the side making a wide stance and allowing your body to dip again.

6. Bring your left leg in to meet your right and stand upright again.

7. Repeat the step to the right, remembering to make a wide low stance allowing your body to dip.

8. Repeat two steps to the left and two steps to the right, alternating each direction until you have achieved 20 steps each way.

This exercise will raise and lower your center of gravity as you move, which will help you to practice the motions that you would need to move between sitting and standing, as well as train your ability to duck away from objects, or gently reach for things in a cupboard. If you find this exercise difficult, it can be performed alongside some kitchen counters so that you are able to reach out and support yourself if you feel that you are going to lose your balance. Try not to look at your feet as you move from side to side; instead, keep your gaze ahead of you. This helps to train the balance center of your brain to understand sideways movement when taken in the context of your forward vision.

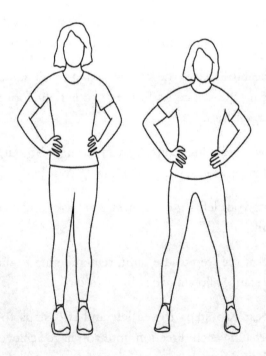

Heel Walks

Areas Targeted: Ankles, knees, hips, and calf muscles; visual input; and proprioception.

1. Stand straight with your feet hip-width apart and your arms at your sides.

2. Lift the balls of both feet off the ground, pointing your toes upwards.

3. Holding your toes off the ground, step forward with your left foot first. Use only your heels to make contact with the floor as you move.

4. Repeat the forward step walking onto your right heel with your toes still in the air.

5. Continue walking one foot in front of the other with only your heels making contact with the floor. Walk this way until you have achieved 20 steps—10 on each foot.

This exercise can be quite demanding, so if you are finding it difficult, you can walk alongside a wall, placing your hand against it for assistance. Keeping your toes pointing upward at all times is the aim. The movements in this exercise can be especially challenging for those who spend a lot of time sitting, and can feel uncomfortable at the back of their calves. At first, you may also feel wobbly. This is fine as long as you do not feel any dizziness. If you experience pain or sudden dizziness, stop immediately and rest.

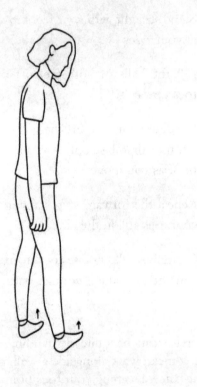

Toe Walks

Areas Targeted: Ankles, knees, hips, and calf muscles; visual input; and proprioception.

1. Stand straight with your feet hip-width apart and your arms at your sides.

2. Rise onto your toes so that the balls of your feet are the only parts of your feet touching the ground.

3. Walk forward, left foot first. Ensure that your heels do not touch the ground as you plant your feet on each step.

4. Repeat the forward step walking onto the toes of your right foot, with your heels still in the air.

5. Continue walking one foot in front of the other with only the balls of your feet making contact with the floor. Walk this way until you have achieved 20 steps—10 on each foot.

If you regularly wear high heels, then this might be a familiar feeling for you. However, with this exercise, you do not have the support of the artificial heel and you will need to work on keeping your heels off the ground. This exercise strengthens the muscles at the back of your calf, which you use to propel yourself forward when walking normally. If you are finding this difficult, you can perform your toe walks alongside a wall so that you can reach your arm out to it for support. This exercise reduces the amount of contact that you have with the floor and challenges your balance centers to keep you steady with a limited area to transfer your weight through. This mimics walking on uneven terrain, stepping down steps, or as mentioned, wearing heels.

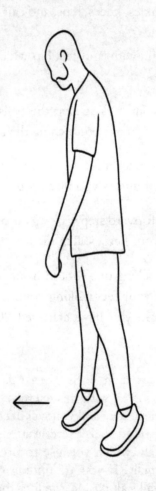

Figure Eight Walking

Areas Targeted: Ankles, knees, hips, abdomen, and back muscles; visual input; coordination; and proprioception—particularly the balance structures in the ear.

1. Place two paper cups on the ground roughly four feet apart.

2. Stand next to the cups so that they form a line traveling away from your side. Choose a location or object in front of you to keep your eyes focused on and continue looking at this spot throughout the exercise.

3. While keeping your eyes focused ahead of you, walk in front of the cup closest to you.

4. Step sideways around the first cup, and then backwards through the gap between the two cups.

5. Step sideways again to travel behind the second cup.

6. Loop around the outside of cup two and then in front of it, now traveling in the opposite direction to that in which you started.

7. Step backwards through the gap between the two cups, and then around the back of the first cup.

8. Continue walking in a figure of eight pattern in front of, between, and behind the two cups until you have completed five circuits around the cups in each direction.

By keeping focused on one spot with your eyes, you are practicing the ability for your brain to understand where your body is in relation to the space around you, as well as developing your ability to maintain your balance through steps in multiple directions. If you are finding this exercise difficult, there are a couple of ways that you can modify it:

- The first is that you can begin by looking in the direction that you are traveling while you walk around the cups rather than maintaining your chosen visual spot. This is a temporary measure and you should aim to be able to complete the figure of eight while looking in only one direction over time.

- If you have no problem maintaining your visual focus but still feel unsteady, you can replace the cups with two dining chairs. This will allow you to reach out and support yourself by holding the backs of the chairs while you are completing the steps. This will increase the size of your figure of eight, so you may also want to reduce the number of circuits that you complete when you begin this way.

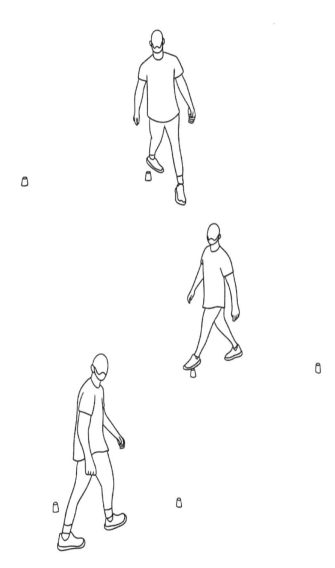

Chapter 7:

Core Exercises

You may have heard people talking about their core muscles before, as it is a very common part of most exercise routines. But something that is less often explained is why these muscles are important for injury prevention, pain reduction, and crucial for maintaining a healthy balance. Your core muscles consist of all the muscles within your pelvis and trunk, supporting your back and stabilizing your posture. These muscles are split into two groups:

1. The inner core, which consists of the muscles that support your spine, some span between your back bones, and others join your pelvis or ribs to your spine, will often be referred to as "core stability exercises."

2. The outer core, which consists of the muscles in your back and around your abdomen that are responsible for the movements generated in your torso, is the one that does the work of bending, twisting, or lifting things. Exercises targeted at this area are often referred to as "core strength exercises."

Having a healthy core system of muscles, both inner and outer, can reduce the onset of chronic back pain, provide your torso with healthy posture, and reduce the likelihood of trips and falls. The balance centers in the brain that rely on proprioception require both core strength and core stability to function correctly to properly understand and control the position of your body in relation to your limbs and anything that is around you.

A Russian Twist

Areas Targeted: Hips, thighs, buttocks, abdomen, back, core, and upper arm muscles; visual input; coordination; and proprioception—particularly the balance structures in the ear.

1. Sit on the floor with your knees bent and your heels touching the ground.

2. Clasp your hands together and lean backward slightly. You need to create enough space between your torso and knees so that you can easily pass your joined hands between them.

3. Twist your torso to the left, placing your hands in the space between your knees and abdomen, then keep twisting to reach your hands out to your left side and towards the ground.

4. Then twist your torso to the right, bringing your hands back to the center and then out to the right towards the ground.

5. Continue twisting, alternating left to right, for 20–40 seconds.

This exercise can be very challenging for anyone who has low core strength, so if you are finding it too difficult in the beginning, don't get discouraged. Adapt the exercise to suit your needs until you are confident enough to perform it fully. To adapt, reduce the amount of lean that you start with. If it is particularly hard for you, you can start by sitting completely upright and twisting from side to side to touch the floor. You will need to lower your knees to be able to do this. Over time, slowly introduce an element of learning and increase the amount a little each time you come back to this exercise.

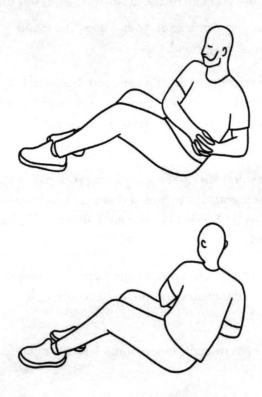

Hollow Crunch

Areas Targeted: Hips, thighs, buttocks, abdomen, back, core, shoulder, and upper arm muscles; visual input; coordination; and proprioception—particularly the balance structures in the ear.

1. Lay on the floor with your legs out straight and your arms by your sides.

2. Raise your arms over your head and bring them back down to the floor above you.

3. Next you need to complete two movements at the same time:

   o Movement one: raise your legs into the air, bending 90 degrees at both your hips and knees, tuck your knees towards your chest.

   o Movement two: lift your arms back over your head and down to your sides, as you bring your arms towards your sides curl your shoulders up off the floor to meet your chest to your knees.

4. Lower your legs and raise your arms above your head.

5. Keep repeating the whole movement for 20–40 seconds.

The aim is to complete the full movement in a slow, controlled manner, avoiding swinging your arms or grabbing onto the sides of your legs to pull yourself forward. Your shoulders and head should raise up off the ground, but you aren't trying to achieve a sit up, instead the goal is to bring your rib cage towards your hips. You can adapt this exercise to make it easier if you are a beginner to core exercises by sitting in a chair and curling your back forwards to bring your ribs down towards your hips.

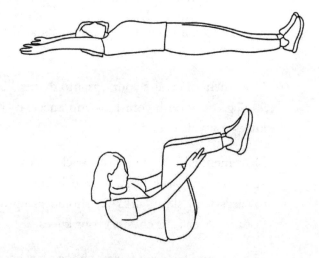

Single Leg Lifts

Areas Targeted: Hips, thighs, buttocks, abdomen, back, core muscles, and proprioception.

1. Lay on the floor with your legs straight and your arms by your sides.

2. Lift your left leg into the air, keeping your knee straight and bending your hip to 90 degrees.

3. Lower your left leg back to the floor.

4. Lift your right leg into the air, keeping your knee straight and bending your hip to 90 degrees.

5. Lower your right leg back to the floor.

6. Continue raising your legs, alternating one at a time for 20–40 seconds.

Tuck your tummy towards the floor while you do this exercise, you don't want to hold your breath, but create a tension in your abdomen. Avoid gripping your hips or legs with your hands while you do this exercise. If it helps you to stop this temptation, you can press your palms flat to the floor instead. Once you are comfortable with this exercise, you can increase the intensity by lifting your head and shoulders off the floor. This creates a mini crunch as you work.

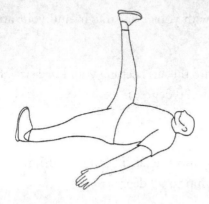

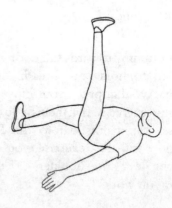

Mountain Climbers

Areas Targeted: Hips, thighs, buttocks, abdomen, back, core, shoulder, and upper arm muscles, coordination, and proprioception.

1. Start by leaning forward on your hands and knees, then straighten your legs out behind you so that the balls of your feet are making contact with the floor.

2. Keep your arms straight at the elbow and your palms flat on the floor at roughly shoulder-width apart.

3. Bend your left leg at the knee and hip, bringing it forward underneath you so that you mimic the starting position of an athletics race.

4. Straighten your left leg again and switch sides.

5. Bend your right leg at the knee and hip, bringing it forwards underneath you.

6. Straighten your right leg again and switch sides.

7. Continue alternating legs for 20–40 seconds.

Be sure to keep your upper back as straight as possible while doing this exercise. A small curl in your lower back is normal, however, as you tuck each knee up towards your chest. Another thing that it is important to avoid is allowing your elbows to twist inwards or outwards, as this can cause unnecessary strain on the joint. The higher you tuck your knees, the more effective this exercise will be.

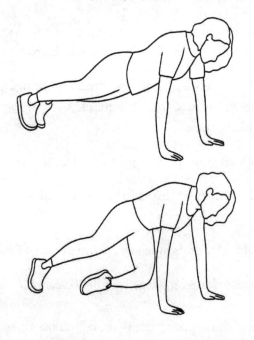

Plank

Areas Targeted: Hips, thighs, buttocks, abdomen, back, core, shoulders, and upper arm muscles, and proprioception.

1. Start by leaning forward on your hands and knees, bend your arms at the elbow and rest your forearms along the floor so that your weight is on your elbows.

2. Straighten your legs out behind you, resting your weight on the balls of your feet.

3. Tuck in your abdomen by gently tensing the muscles and holding this position for 20–40 seconds.

4. Exit the hold position by bending your legs at the knees and hips to rest your weight through your knees, and then sit up.

The plank is a challenging task for any beginner to core exercise, so you can adapt it to yourself by reducing the amount of time that you hold the position. Start with as low as 10 seconds and gradually increase your hold as you become more practiced. Once you are comfortable achieving 40-second holds, you can increase the intensity of this exercise by bending your knees to take a short rest and then holding again for up to three repetitions. I prefer to split the exercise into reps rather than increase the length of hold past 40 seconds, as a longer hold increases the temptation to bend at the hips, which reduces its effectiveness and activates the wrong muscles.

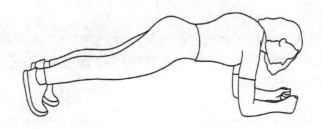

Side Plank

Areas Targeted: Hips, thighs, buttocks, abdomen, back, core, shoulder, and upper arm muscles, and proprioception.

1. Lay on your left side on the floor with your legs straight.

2. Lift your torso off the floor with one arm, leaning your weight through your elbow with your forearm lying flat across the floor pointing in front of you.

3. Lift your hips upwards to create a straight line with your body.

4. Tuck in your abdomen by gently tensing the abdominal muscles and holding this position for 20–40 seconds.

5. Exit this position by first lowering your hips back to the ground and then your shoulders.

6. Switch sides and repeat on your right side, holding for 20–40 seconds.

It is important to remember to tuck in your abdomen as activating these muscles will provide support to your lower back while you perform this exercise as well as increase the effectiveness of this position. Avoid the temptation to allow your hips to dip, creating a curve in the line of your body. Instead, aim to keep an imaginary line from your head, along your spine, and down your legs to the floor as straight as possible. As with the plank, I recommend adding extra repetitions with rests in between if you feel confident in increasing the intensity of your side planks.

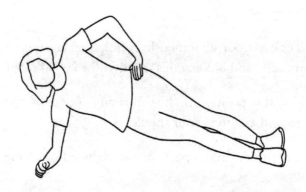

Chapter 8:

Vestibular Exercises

What Is Vestibular Exercise?

Vestibular exercises are a unique sub-set of exercises targeted specifically at training the balance centers in your brain and nervous system. The goal of these exercises is to challenge your brain to reinterpret its memory of how balance works for you. Over time, vestibular routines will reprogram the balance center of your brain to compensate for any injuries, abnormalities in the nervous system, or other contributors to poor balance that you may have. The overall outcome of these routines is that you will experience improved spells of dizziness, improved posture and stability within each posture, improved stability of your gaze while moving, and ultimately an improved quality of life due to gaining confidence in yourself that you can move about safely and without fear of falling.

Vestibular exercises will focus on training your gaze stability, hand-eye coordination, and correcting any compensations that you may be making due to an existing ailment in your balance centers; reducing the effects of aging on your ability to balance; and improving your ability to remain stable with multi-directional movements.

Each exercise will challenge the point at which you experience dizziness. For that reason, it is normal to feel some dizziness when you start. You will then work on that point of activating dizziness to push it back and become more confident. However, if you experience anything more than mild dizziness or discomfort, you should stop immediately and consult your health practitioner. Like any exercise aimed at strengthening muscles, vestibular exercises work best when consistently repeated and gradually increased in intensity. In the beginning, you may want to be sure that you practice these exercises with surfaces nearby that you can hold onto for support if you feel overwhelmed. If you have an existing balance disorder such as vertigo, you may also want to start these exercises with someone else present to help you.

ZigZag Walking

Areas Targeted: Hips, thighs, buttocks, abdomen, and back muscles; visual input; coordination, and proprioception.

1. Start in an area where you have plenty of space in front of and to the side of you.

2. Stand with your feet hip width apart and your hands at your sides.

3. Choose a location on the wall opposite you, or an item at the far end of the room and keep your gaze fixed on that location or item.

4. Walk forward in a diagonal line to your left.

5. Once you reach the opposite side of your exercise space, change directions so that you are walking in a diagonal line to your right. Remember to keep your gaze fixed on your chosen location while you are walking, this will result in your head turning to the side as you walk.

6. Continue switching directions until you have completed five diagonal walks in each direction.

If you have limited space, you can still do this exercise by completing one or two diagonal walks and then going back to your starting position to do more. The key to this exercise being successful is to maintain your gaze position throughout. You will be training your body to understand how movement feels when it is occurring in a direction at odds with your vision and to strengthen its ability to maintain posture and stability when doing so. Don't be afraid to take a rest in between each zigzag set if you need to. You want to avoid pushing yourself until you are dizzy or faint.

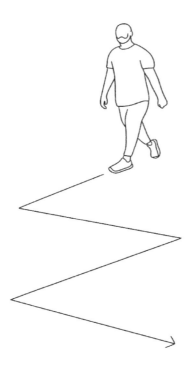

Eyes Side to Side

Areas Targeted: Facial muscles around the eyes, visual input, and proprioception.

1. Stand straight with your feet hip-width apart for stability.

2. Hold your arms still and point your head directly forward.

3. Look to your left as far as you can move your eyes only.

4. Then switch directions and look to the right as far as you can without moving your head.

5. Keep alternating the direction that you move your eyes until you have achieved 15 sets of looking in each direction.

If you find this exercise difficult or have a history of falls, you may wish to begin by training your eye movements while sitting and gradually move on to being able to complete this while standing. You should aim to keep your head facing forward throughout this exercise to train your balance center to interpret your surroundings and understand that movement of the gaze doesn't equate to movement of the body.

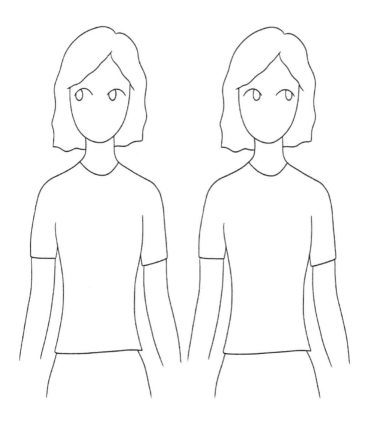

Eyes Up and Down

Areas Targeted: Facial muscles around the eyes, visual input, and proprioception.

1. Stand straight with your feet hip-width apart for stability.

2. Hold your arms still and point your head directly forward.

3. Look upwards as far as you can move your eyes only.

4. Then switch directions and look downwards as far as you can without moving your head.

5. Keep alternating the direction that you move your eyes until you have achieved 15 sets of looking up and down.

As with the eyes side to side exercise, if you are a beginner or have previously experienced falls, you may wish to start this exercise in a seated position first. Once you are more confident, you can build up to doing this in a standing position. Looking up can be particularly difficult if you suffer from vertigo or other balance disorders linked to the balance center. If this is the case for you, you may want to conduct these exercises in front of a kitchen counter so that you can hold onto it for support.

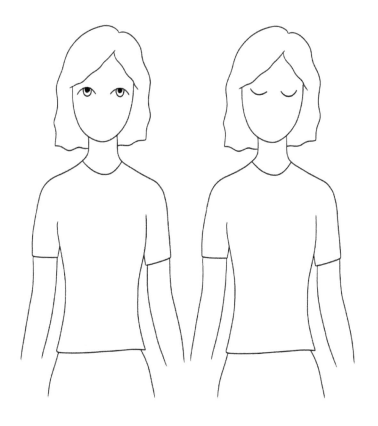

In and Out

Areas Targeted: Facial muscles around the eye, shoulder, and upper arm muscles, visual input, coordination, and proprioception.

1. Stand straight with your feet hip-width apart for stability.

2. Point your head directly forward.

3. Lift one arm and use your pointer finger to point towards the ceiling.

4. Focus your gaze on the tip of your finger while your hand is at full arm's length.

5. Slowly bring your hand toward your face until your pointer finger is touching your nose. Keep your gaze fixed on the tip of your finger as it moves towards you.

6. Then switch directions and slowly move your hand away from your face until it is once again at full arm's length. Keep your gaze fixed on the tip of your finger as it moves away from you.

7. Keep alternating the direction that you move your hand until you have achieved 15 sets of focus on your pointer finger as it moves towards and away from you.

Remember to move your arm in a slow, steady line to and from your face. If you do this too quickly, it can increase the tendency to only focus on the beginning and end positions of your finger, forgetting all the distance in between. If you have any existing visual impairments that you have been prescribed glasses to correct, you will want to be sure that you have these on during this exercise to avoid causing a headache.

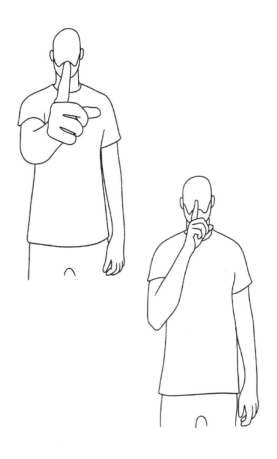

Head Up and Down

Areas Targeted: Neck and back muscles, visual input, and proprioception—particularly the balance structures in the ear.

1. Stand with your feet hip-width apart and your arms still at your sides.

2. The starting position for your head should be facing forward.

3. Tilt your head back to look up at the ceiling.

4. Then, bring your head back to its natural resting position.

5. Tilt your head downward, bringing your chin to your chest and looking down at the floor.

6. Then, bring your head back to its natural resting position.

7. Continue alternating between looking up to the ceiling and down to the floor until you have achieved 15 sets of this movement.

Be sure to look all the way up to the ceiling and then all the way down to the floor, allowing your head to follow the direction of your gaze, rather than moving your head first and then adjusting your vision. If you are finding this exercise difficult, you can adapt it by halving the distance that you move your head as you look up or down when you first begin. You can then slowly increase the distance that you look as you become more confident. If you have a history of falls, you may wish to perform this exercise while sitting in a chair until you are more confident, particularly while looking upwards.

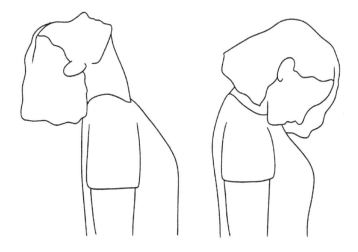

Head Side to Side

Areas Targeted: Neck and muscles, visual input, and proprioception—particularly the balance structures in the ear.

1. Stand with your feet hip-width apart and your arms still at your sides.

2. The starting position for your head should be facing forward.

3. Turn your head to look to your left as far as possible.

4. Then, bring your head back to its natural resting position.

5. Turn your head to look to your right as far as possible.

6. Then, bring your head back to its natural resting position.

7. Continue alternating directions until you have achieved 15 sets of looking left and right.

Aim to keep your motions smooth and steady as you change directions. Be sure to allow your head to follow the direction of your gaze, rather than moving your head first and then adjusting your vision. When you look from left to right, look as far in each direction as you can without twisting your torso. If you are finding this difficult or have a history of falls, you may wish to practice this exercise in a chair before you perform it while standing.

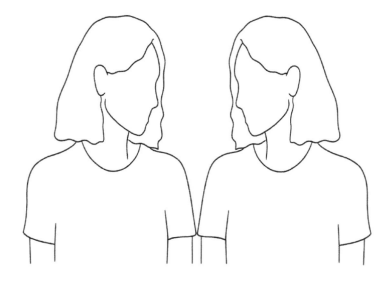

Sitting to Standing With Rotation

Areas Targeted: Legs and core muscles, visual input, coordination, and proprioception—particularly the balance structures in the ear.

1. Sit in a chair with your feet hip width apart.

2. Lean forward and plant your weight through your feet, then stand up.

3. Walk in a circle on the spot to your left:

    ○   Start by turning your left foot out to your side and transferring your weight to it.

    ○   Move your right foot next to your left, following through to turn your body.

    ○   Keep stepping this way until you have completed a full circle. This should be approximately 4–5 steps.

    ○   Once you have turned a full circle and you once again have your back to the chair, sit back down.

4. Repeat steps 1–4 until you have achieved five full sit-to-stand and rotations.

This exercise combines several skills that you may need to practice separately if you find it difficult to get into and out of chairs. If you are finding it particularly difficult, try placing your hands on your legs above your knees and pushing down through them as you stand. Alternatively, you could also swap your chair for one with arms built in and push down through those instead of placing your hands on your legs. Remember, though, if you switch your chair, that it still needs to have a solid base and back. Avoid using a recliner. It is normal when you begin to feel slightly dizzy while rotating your body on the spot. However, if this becomes disorienting or you feel lightheaded stop immediately. You should use extra caution in this exercise if you have vertigo or similar pre-existing balance disorders.

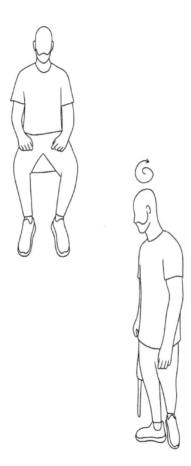

Ball Toss Head Height

Areas Targeted: Shoulder and arm muscles, visual input, coordination, reaction times, and proprioception.

For this exercise, you will need a small ball, like a ping-pong ball or a juggling ball.

1. Stand with your feet hip-width apart.

2. Lift both arms so that your elbows are bent and your hands are at the level of your face.

3. Hold the ball in your left hand then throw it from left to right in front of you, catching it with your right hand.

4. Throw the ball back from your right hand across in front of you, catching it with your left hand.

5. Keep throwing the ball from left to right and back again until you have achieved 20 sets.

Aim to keep your head facing forwards throughout this exercise. Try not to follow the direction that the ball travels. This exercise will help to develop your hand eye coordination, along with developing your brain's ability to locate the position of your hands precisely and rapidly. Don't worry if you find this exercise difficult at first. It is normal for this to require practice, and you will need patience to build up to 20 successful catches of the ball.

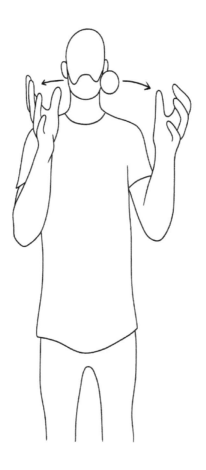

Ball Toss Between the Legs

Areas Targeted: Hips, thighs, buttocks, abdomen, back, core, and arm muscles; visual input; coordination; reaction times; and proprioception.

For this exercise, you will need a small ball, like a ping-pong ball or a juggling ball.

1. Stand with your feet hip-width apart.

2. Step forward on your left foot, and bend your knees slightly.

3. Lean forward so that your hands are below the level of your left thigh.

4. Hold the ball in your left hand then throw it from left to right between your legs, catching it with your right hand.

5. Throw the ball back from your right hand, under your leg, catching it with your left hand.

6. Keep throwing the ball from left to right and back again until you have achieved 10 sets.

7. Return to standing with your feet hip-width apart and take a short break if needed.

8. Step forward on your right foot, and bend your knees slightly.

9. Lean forward so that your hands are below the level of your left thigh.

10. Then repeat the process of throwing the ball from left to right underneath the front leg until you have achieved another 10 sets.

This exercise tests your balance from both a physical aspect, in your muscles' ability to hold the stance required, and a balance center perspective to train your coordination. If you are finding this exercise difficult, you can drop the knee of the back leg to the floor so that your shin is resting along the ground and your front leg is bent at 90 degrees at both the knee and hip. You can also practice the hand motions without the ball and then reintroduce the ball toss once you are confident that you can safely hold the stance required.

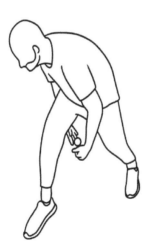

Chapter 9:

Advanced Balance Exercises

The exercises contained in this Chapter are very challenging. They combine multiple aspects of balance training and may need to be practiced in smaller sections before you put them all together as you become more confident. Remember to practice each exercise with caution. Training may feel uncomfortable, but it should never be painful. If you feel any pain, lightheadedness, or disorientation, then you should stop and consult with your primary physician or other health professional. Consider keeping a chair nearby or working out next to a kitchen counter that you can hold onto if you feel unstable at any point. You may also want to have someone with you to lend a hand if you become particularly dizzy.

Around the World

Areas Targeted: Ankles, knees, hips, thighs, buttocks, abdomen, back, and core muscles; visual input; coordination; and proprioception—particularly the balance structures in the ear.

1. Stand with your feet hip-width apart.

2. Bend your left leg at the knee to dip your body towards the ground as you reach your right foot forward and touch your right foot to the floor.

3. Straighten your legs and bring your right foot back in to join your left.

4. Bend your left leg again, this time reaching your right leg out to your right side and touch your foot to the floor.

5. Straighten your legs and bring your right foot back in to join your left.

6. Bend your left leg once more, reaching your right leg out behind you and touching your foot to the floor.

7. Straighten your legs and bring your right foot back in to join your left.

8. Keep your left leg straight and cross your right leg over in front of it, to tap your right foot to the ground at your left side.

9. Uncross your legs and bring your right foot back in to join your left.

10. Repeat this pattern until you have reached all four directions three times.

11. Once the three sets are completed, switch the leg that you are using to reach out with to your left leg.

12. Bend your right leg at the knee to dip your body towards the ground as you reach your left foot forward and touch your left foot to the floor.

13. Straighten your legs and bring your left foot back in to join your right.

14. Bend your right leg again, this time reaching your left leg out to your left side and bringing your foot to the floor.

15. Straighten your legs and bring your left foot back in to join your right.

16. Bend your right leg once more, reaching your left leg out behind you and touching your foot to the floor.

17. Straighten your legs and bring your left foot back in to join your right.

18. Keep your right leg straight and cross your left leg over in front of it, to tap your left foot to the ground at your right side.

19. Uncross your legs and bring your left foot back in to join your left.

20. Repeat this pattern until you have reached all four directions three times.

If you are finding it difficult to complete this exercise, you can reduce the distance from the body that you reach with the foot that you are moving in each direction. This will reduce the pressure on your weight bearing leg as you bend the knee. Similarly, if you have been practicing for a few weeks and are safely completing the full cycle with confidence, you can reach further away to dial up the difficulty of this exercise.

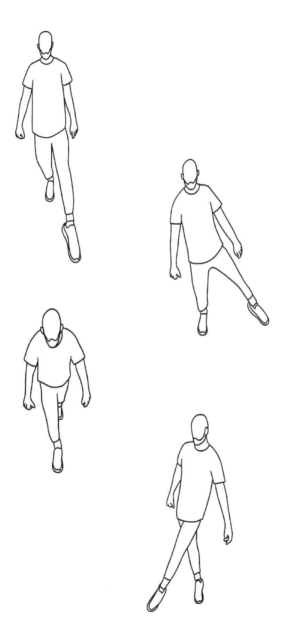

Tree Pose

Areas Targeted: Feet, ankles, knees, hips, thighs, buttocks, abdomen, back, and core muscles; visual input; coordination; and proprioception.

1. Stand with your feet hip-width apart and your arms at your sides.

2. Lift your left foot, bending your leg at the knee.

3. Place the sole of your left foot against the inside of your right leg with your toes pointing downward.

4. Hold this position for 20–60 seconds.

5. Place your left foot back on the ground.

6. Then, lift your right foot, bending your leg at the knee.

7. Place the sole of your right foot against the inside of your left leg with your toes pointing downward.

8. Hold this position for 20–60 seconds.

The goal when doing this exercise is to place the sole of your lifted foot above the knee of the opposite leg and keep your arms at your sides. If you are finding it difficult to get into the correct position, you can adapt the exercise by lowering your foot. The lower your foot, the easier the exercise will become. However, be sure never to place your foot directly against the opposite knee, to avoid placing unnecessary pressure on that joint. You can also raise your arms out to your sides so that they are level with your shoulders to help you maintain your balance until you are confident enough to keep them at your sides. In the beginning, aiming for a 20-second hold may seem like a challenge, and that is fine. You can increase the length of your pose each time you practice until you gradually reach 60 seconds.

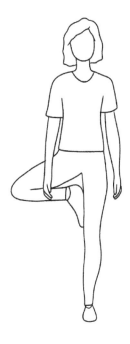

Front Scale

Areas Targeted: Ankles, knees, hips, thighs, buttocks, abdomen, back, core, shoulder, and upper arm muscles, visual input, coordination, and proprioception.

1. Stand with your feet hip-width apart and your arms at your sides.

2. Lift your left leg, bending only at the hip and hold it straight out in front of you.

3. Lift your arms out to your sides to help you maintain your balance.

4. Hold this position for 20–60 seconds.

5. Lower your left leg to the floor and switch sides.

6. Lift your right leg, bending only at the hip and hold it straight out in front of you.

7. Lift your arms out to your sides to help you maintain your balance.

8. Hold this position for 20–60 seconds.

Start by aiming to hold your pose for 20 seconds at a time. Then, gradually increase the length of time that you hold your position as you become more practiced, until you can confidently reach a 60-second hold. Once you are safely achieving 60-second holds on both legs, you can increase the intensity of the exercise by lowering your arms and aiming to achieve the hold with both arms resting at your sides. Conversely, if you are finding this exercise difficult, you can keep a chair at your side and reach out to hold it until your balance is strong enough for you to no longer need the support.

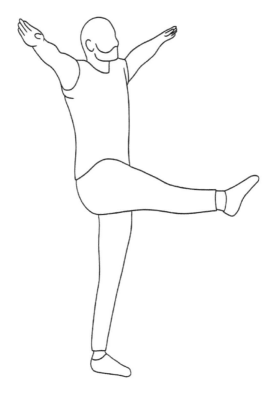

Back Scale

Areas Targeted: Ankles, knees, hips, thighs, buttocks, abdomen, back, and core muscles; visual input; coordination; and proprioception—particularly the balance structures in the ear.

1. Stand with your feet hip-width apart.

2. Lift your left leg out behind you and lean forward until you create a horizontal line along your back and down the length of your leg that is parallel to the floor.

3. Spread your arms out to the sides to help you maintain your balance.

4. Hold this pose for 20–60 seconds.

5. Lower your left leg back to the floor and stand upright, then switch sides.

6. Lift your right leg out behind you and lean forward until you create a horizontal line along your back and down the length of your leg that is parallel to the floor.

7. Spread your arms out to the sides to help you maintain your balance.

8. Hold this pose for 20–60 seconds.

As with the front lean, begin by setting yourself a target of 20 seconds for your hold time. Once you are comfortable with achieving this time on both sides, you can begin increasing your hold until you reach 60 seconds on each side. After you have achieved a full 60-second hold and are confident that you can safely begin to adapt to this exercise, you can make it more difficult by pulling your arms in toward your sides or holding them in front of your chest with your elbows bent. If you are finding this exercise difficult, you can keep a chair nearby so that you can hold it back while you practice, until you are safely able to hold the pose without needing the extra support.

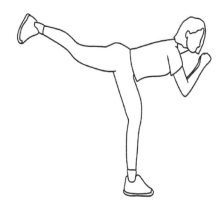

Chapter 10:

Different Tools for Balance

As with any form of exercise, you can assist your balance training by making use of specialist equipment. This doesn't mean that the equipment is difficult to source or that it must be prescribed by a health professional, but that it is designed specifically for the purpose of improving your ability to balance and creating a healthier balance center. There are many forms of equipment available on the market today, and it can be intimidating to search for something that suits your needs. In this Chapter, I break down four kinds of specialty equipment that I believe are the most effective in enhancing balance training routines.

Balance Board

Balance boards can be used to replicate a variety of situations where your balance will be tested. You use balance boards by placing them soft side down and standing on top, then adapting your movements each time the board moves to stay upright. By putting your body into these positions, you can train your ability to react appropriately to this kind of stimulus and improve your balance for many everyday activities. Balance boards usually consist of a soft base such as a rubber or plastic dome and a hard top surface that extends away from the base that you can stand on while you exercise. The boards are usually plastic or wood for strength so that they can easily hold your weight and are often used in rehabilitation classes following injuries.

While they started as a rehabilitation tool in therapy settings, there are many types of balance boards available on the market today for use at home:

1. **Traditional balance board**: Usually a wooden top surface with a soft cylindrical bottom that allows movement in a linear direction.

2. **Wobble board**: Can be plastic or wood but usually include a tough grip surface on top and a half ball shape underneath that gives free movement in 360 degrees around the center.

3. **Electronic balance boards**: These are plastic and usually consist of two flat surfaces separated by bars and push buttons that provide movement and resistance. They will provide feedback on your performance through a visual display, these can be expensive, but there are also some available that are designed to function with gaming consoles.

4. **Lateral slide boards**: These boards consist of two flat surfaces separated by bars. Unlike the electronic boards, these don't provide resistance and only have end bumpers to prevent the top board slipping off entirely. These are very challenging and are not recommended for beginners.

5. **Standing desk balance board**: These can provide linear or 360-degree movement but are generally a bit stiffer than other boards so that they are less mobile and able to be used for longer periods of time.

Using a balance board is an advanced way of pushing your balance training, so it is important that you start any exercise with this tool near to a surface you can hold for stability or with another person for support, until you become more adept at using the balance board. The movement of the balance board can be unpredictable, especially when you first start using it while your natural reaction to maintain your center of balance is likely compromised. The board will cause you to continually make corrections in your posture to remain upright, so it can be labor intensive. For this reason, you should begin with short sessions, aiming to remain balanced for 20–60 seconds. Once you achieve this safely, you can increase the amount of time that you spend using the balance board to suit your own goals. Some people even use them for long periods of time in front of a standing desk while they work.

After you become confident in standing on a balance board safely, you can challenge yourself by completing exercises while using the board. You can add in things like a squat or torso lean in any direction. You can also introduce the *Ball Toss Head Height* exercise featured in Chapter 8. There are many ideas easily found online for adapting your balance board routine. Try experimenting to find a challenge that you enjoy and that suits your own personal balance goals.

Bosu Ball

Bosu Balls were designed in 1999 by David Weck and the name stands for *both sides utilized* (Mead, 2022). It is a semi-sphere that resembles half of an exercise ball with a flat surface that does not significantly extend past the diameter of that ball half. When used with the flat side up, the bosu ball creates an unstable surface that can be utilized in the same way as a balance board, but when used with the flat side down, the ball becomes much more versatile. The flat surface against the ground creates a stable surface that isn't going to move while you exercise with it, but more uniquely, the upper curved surface, which is full of air like an exercise ball, provides a cushioned surface that you can use to train your balance while simultaneously lessening the load on your joints as you move through your exercises.

The curved surface of the bosu ball can be used to provide support for back and abdominal stretches that allow you to safely stretch further than you may be able to while sitting or standing. To take advantage of this, for example, you can train your core strength by laying on your side, placing your hips on top–but near to the edge–of the curved surface, creating an anchor for yourself against the floor by placing your legs roughly shoulder-width apart on the ground in front of each other. You can then lower your upper body over the curve of the bosu ball so that your shoulders move towards the floor, lifting your shoulders back up to create a curve in your spine in the opposite direction towards the ceiling. Complete 15–20 of these stretch combinations on each side. The ball can be used in this way for abdomen stretches; moving your shoulders towards the floor while laying on your back, combined with a mini crunch to lift your shoulders back up, or as a support for your feet while doing calf stretches—there are multiple videos available online giving inspiration for using the bosu ball as a stretching aid.

In addition to the advantages that the bosu ball brings in terms of active stretching, it can also be used flat side down to enhance your balance training. Standing on top of the curved surface barefoot can improve the way your brain processes feedback from the feet to make corrections in posture necessary to keep you stable. Another advantage to working on the bosu ball barefoot is that it will give you an opportunity to strengthen muscles in the foot that you wouldn't ordinarily use while wearing shoes but that play an important role in a healthy ability to balance. After some practice, once you are confident that you can stand on the curved surface safely, you can introduce some of the standing exercises in Chapter 5 while on the bosu ball. Exercises like toe taps, heel taps, and forward leans can be particularly effective when paired with this tool, as the bosu ball encourages activation of your whole core while progressing through them.

Balance Pad

Balance pads are square sponge or gel pads–usually around three inches thick–that create an unstable surface which can be stood on while exercising to encourage activation of muscles needed for stability. Unlike balance boards, they don't produce large movements that require a lot of adaptation in your posture to master. Because of this, they are great for beginners or anyone with a history of falls, ankle rolls, or pre-existing balance disorders. Balance pads are particularly useful for strengthening the muscles around your ankles and knees, though they also force you to practice your ability to process feedback from your feet to make body wide corrections to remain upright.

As a beginner's tool, a great way to get started is to stand with both feet on the pad and close one eye to see how this affects how stable your body feels. Do practice closing each eye and comparing them to see if you notice a difference between the left and right. Do you feel like you need to employ more corrections to your posture on one side than the other? It isn't unusual to feel a disparity between the two, especially if you have injured one leg or ankle in the past. For people who experience a lot of balance difficulties, this alone can be a challenging exercise, but once it is mastered, the balance pad can be used in many standing exercises to work the balance center and muscles simultaneously.

Some of my favorite exercise adaptations for the balance pad include:

- **Toe or heel raises; Chapter 5**: Stand central on the balance pad and perform the toe and heel raise to challenge your ankles and core.

- **High Knee Marches on the Spot; Chapter 6**: March on top of the balance pad to strengthen your legs and hips.

- **Sidesteps; Chapter 6**: Start on the bare floor next to the balance pad and sidestep onto it, then sidestep again off the other side. Practice both directions. This will encourage your balance center to process changing ground types as you move.

- **Russian twists; Chapter 7**: Sit on the balance pad to perform your twists. This will increase the work that your core must do to remain in the required pose and will increase the intensity of this exercise.

- **Plank or side plank; Chapter 7**: Rest your arms on the balance pad while doing these exercises to challenge your core in maintaining a straight spine.

- **Tree Pose, Chapter 9**: This exercise adaptation shouldn't be attempted by beginners. Be sure that you are confident in performing the tree pose on the bare ground before attempting to use the balance pad here. stand on top of the balance pad to practice this pose, try to keep the foot that you are standing on as close as possible to the center of the pad. This will challenge your balance center and whole body to maintain a stable position.

Stability Ball

The stability ball is an air-filled ball that comes in a variety of sizes and is also known as the "exercise ball," "swiss ball," or "physio ball." Like other equipment, it was initially used as a rehabilitation tool but has since been adopted by several gyms and is an inexpensive home exercise addition. Stability balls are the most readily available and accessible tool in this Chapter. They aren't recommended for standing but can replace a chair in any seated exercise to increase the effectiveness of that workout. Stability balls are hailed for their ability to improve posture and have even been taken into offices in place of regular chairs to facilitate the wellness of workers.

There is more than just good posture to be gained from the stability ball. However, like the other tools listed here, it forces your body to process feedback about its position and constantly adjust to remain stable, becoming an effective balance training aid. The key area of the body trained by the stability ball is the core. Muscles in the lower back are activated immediately to keep you in place when you sit on it. Additional benefits include reduced load on the joints in the same way that the bosu board cushions the body, improved reaction time, reduced back pain, and improved confidence in mobility.

Conclusion

Physical well-being necessitates listening to what you already know, and then taking it seriously enough to act accordingly. When you wake up and feel the impulse to arch your back, stretch and exhale with a loud sigh, for God's sake, do it. –Darrell Calkins

They say that the best time to start anything new was yesterday, but the second-best time is today. Now that you have access to a bank of well-rounded balanced targeted exercises, you can build your muscle coordination, improve your proprioception, strengthen your core, and feel confident in getting back out there to enjoy life without fear of falling.

Remember to set a regular time that suits you and commit to your routine. Consistent balance practice is key to really making the most of your exercises. You don't need to slog through the whole book every day; instead, complete your warm-up and choose ten exercises that will total around 15 minutes per day. Make sure you switch up your chosen exercises each time you workout to keep things enjoyable, and make sure you train your whole body. Preparing a plan of exercise rotations in advance can help to make sure that you don't miss out on any important tasks. This is why I created my weekly planner and made it available to you for free! I want to give you all the tools you need to succeed.

To receive your complimentary copy now, please visit *www.robertbalazs.com.*

This is also what drove me to create a book that is fully illustrated and to provide videos of each exercise being performed from start to finish. Everyone has a different way of learning and taking in information, so I wanted to make these exercises as accessible as possible no matter which style of learning suits you best.

To get your video companion playlist, please visit *www.tinyurl.com/Rob-Balazs*.

The exercise adaptations in this book are intended to make the exercises feasible for all ability levels, whether you have existing balance disorders or are recovering from an injury, or you consider yourself generally healthy but have noticed that your coordination isn't what it used to be. Remember, there are always ways to make the exercises easier on you when you are feeling out of your depth. You don't need to feel like balance training is too complicated or difficult for you. On the flip side, once you have been practicing for some time, you may feel like you want a bit more of a challenge, then it's time to embrace the advanced exercises and examine tools for balance training so that you can push yourself while working out.

We all know that you will be more disappointed by the things you didn't do than by the ones you did. Go for it! Enjoy every second of this journey and come back with a ton of amazing memories. –Unknown

You can look forward to better reaction times, coordination, and improved stability. So, what are you waiting for? There is no time like the present. Start your weekly planner and get on your way to a healthier balance today.

No matter where you start in ability level, I can't wait to see where your balance training journey takes you and would love to hear your feedback via reviews.

To leave a review, scan the QR code at the beginning of the book with your mobile phone and click on the book. Once you have clicked on the book, you will be able to find the button to leave a review. If you don't have a smartphone able to scan the QR code, you can also access the reviews by searching for the book title again on Amazon.

References

Balance Problems: Basic Facts. (2022). AGS Health in Aging Foundation. https://www.healthinaging.org/a-z-topic/balance-problems/basic-facts

Back To Motion Physical Therapy. (n.d.). Importance of Balance Training for Seniors - Back To Motion. *Denver Physical Therapy. Back to Motion Physical Therapy.* https://backtomotion.net/importance-of-balance-training-for-seniors/

Bhupathiraju, S. (2022, April 7). 9 Best Vestibular Exercises. *Styles At Life.* https://stylesatlife.com/articles/vestibular-exercises/

Brennan, D. (2021, March 18). What Causes Balance Issues in Older Adults. *WebMD.* http://https_www.webmd.com/?url=https%3A%2F%2Fwww.webmd.com%2Fhealthy-aging%2Fwhat-causes-balance-issues-in-older-adults

Carroll, J. (2005, December 6). Regular Exercise: Who's Getting It? *Gallup News.* https://news.gallup.com/poll/20314/Regular-Exercise-Whos-Getting-It.aspx

Centers for Disease Control and Prevention. (2021, August 6). Facts About Falls. *Centers for Disease Control and Prevention.* https://www.cdc.gov/falls/facts.html

Dillon, C. F., Gu, Q., Hoffman, H. J., & Ko, C.-W. (2010, April). Vision, Hearing, Balance, and Sensory Impairment in Americans Aged 70 Years and Over: United States, 1999–2006. *NCHS Data Brief*, 31, 1-8.

Edwards, D. (2019, August 19). The Top 8 Benefits of Balance Training. *Primal Play*. https://www.primalplay.com/blog/8-benefits-of-balance-exercises

Elderly Fall Prevention. (2022). Choosing the Right Walking Aids. *Elderly Fall Prevention*. https://elderlyfallprevention.com/assistive-devices/walking-aids/

Elflein, J. (2021, February 16). • Prevalence of moderate or severe vision impairment by age and gender worldwide 2020. *Statista*. https://www.statista.com/statistics/1238083/prevalence-moderate-severe-vision-impairment-by-age-gender/

Fitness Drum. (2021, April 26). Balance Pad Exercises That Will Work Wonders For Your Stability and Body Control. *Fitness Drum*. https://fitnessdrum.com/balance-pad-exercises/

Fox, R. (2022, April 30). Why Balance Is So Important For Seniors (and How To Improve Yours). *Silver Fox Fitness*. https://gentlestrengthexercises.com/why-balance-is-so-important-for-seniors/

Freedom Care. (2020, June 24). Why Senior Citizens Should Perform Balance Exercises. *FreedomCare*.

https://www.freedomcareny.com/posts/why-should-senior-citizens-perform-balance-exercises

Gaspari Nutrition. (2019, July 10). What Are The Pros & Cons of BOSU Balls? *Gaspari Nutrition.* https://gasparinutrition.com/blogs/fitness-facts/what-are-the-pros-cons-of-bosu-balls

Han, B. I., Song, H. S., & Kim, J. S. (2011, December 29). Vestibular Rehabilitation Therapy: Review of Indications, Mechanisms, and Key Exercises. *Journal of Clinical Neurology, 7*(4), 184-196. 10.3988/jcn.2011.7.4.184

Huffman, M. (2015, May 14). Use of walking aids jumps 50% in 10 years. *ConsumerAffairs.com.* https://www.consumeraffairs.com/news/use-of-walking-aids-jumps-50-in-10-years-051415.html

Kinetix Physical Therapy. (2022). The Connection Between Core Strength and Better Balance. *Kinetix Physical Therapy.* https://kinetixpt.com/the-connection-between-core-strength-and-better-balance/

Konrad, H. R., Giradi, M., & Helfert, R. (1999, September). Balance and Aging. *The Laryngoscope, 109*(9), 1454-60. 10.1097/00005537-199909000-00019

Larsen, E. (n.d.). 4 Proven Benefits of Stability Ball Exercises: Science And Facts | FITNESS. *HomeTrainingHero.* https://www.hometraininghero.com/benefits-stability-ball-exercises-science-behind-effectiveness/

Leaf Group Ltd. (2022). Why You Should Train With a Balance Board and How to Get Started. *Livestrong.com.*

https://www.livestrong.com/article/34421-balance-board-benefits/

Mayo Clinic. (2020, August 29). Core exercises: Why you should strengthen your core muscles. *Mayo Clinic.* https://www.mayoclinic.org/healthy-lifestyle/fitness/in-depth/core-exercises/art-20044751

McKeon, P. O., & Hartel, J. (2008, May-June). Systematic review of postural control and lateral ankle instability, part II: is balance training clinically effective? *Journal of Athletic Training, 43*(3), 305-15. 10.4085/1062-6050-43.3.305

McKeon, P. O., Ingersoll, C. D., Kerrigan, D. C., Saliba, E., Bennett, B. C., & Hartel, J. (2008, October). Balance training improves function and postural control in those with chronic ankle instability. *Medicine and Science in Sports and Exercise, 40*(10), 1810-9. 10.1249/MSS.0b013e31817e0f92

Mead, T. (2022). What Is A Bosu Ball And How To Use It. *Alternative Daily.* https://www.thealternativedaily.com/how-to-use-a-bosu-ball/

National Institute on Aging. (2022, June 16). Prevent Falls and Fractures | National Institute on Aging. *National Institute on Aging.* https://www.nia.nih.gov/health/prevent-falls-and-fractures

North Central Surgical Center. (2016, March 10). The benefits of exercising with a stability ball. *North Central Surgical Center.* https://www.northcentralsurgical.com/blog/the-benefits-of-exercising-with-a-stability-ball-54.html

Rettner, R. (2016, July 8). Everything You Need to Know About Balance Exercise. *Live Science*. https://www.livescience.com/55321-balance-exercise.html

Smith, E. (2015, January 5). The Benefits of a Bosu Ball. *American Home Fitness*. https://americanhomefitness.com/blogs/news/the-benefits-of-a-bosu-ball

Techno Gym. (n.d.). Balance Pad: Exercises for Your Workout. *Technogym*. https://www.technogym.com/us/newsroom/balance-pad-exercises-workout/

University of Mississippi. (n.d.). Vestibular (Balance) Exercises. *University of Mississippi Medical Center*. https://www.umc.edu/Healthcare/ENT/Patient-Handouts/Adult/Otology/Vestibular_Exercises.html

U.S. Department of Health & Human Services. (2022, June 3). How much physical activity do older adults need? | *Physical Activity. CDC*. https://www.cdc.gov/physicalactivity/basics/older_adults/index.htm

Stretching For Seniors

Key Exercises for 50+ That Will
Improve Your Posture, Relieve
Joint And Back Pain, Setting You
Up For A Healthier Future

Robert Balazs

Introduction

I don't let my age define me, but the side effects are getting harder to ignore.
-Unknown

Aging is a normal part of human life, and while unavoidable, there are things that can be done to relieve the aches and pains that accompany it. You can, to a certain extent, even reverse the decline in your flexibility and muscle mass and improve your energy levels.

As we age it is common for the number of us taking part in regular physical activity to decline, especially after retirement for those of us who have reached that milestone. Injuries sustained throughout our lives and long-term bad habits that we develop over time, can damage our joints and ruin our posture. Bad posture also has the knock-on effect of making walking more difficult, or experiencing pain even when at rest.

Understandably though, when we are in pain or suffering from stiff joints, it can be difficult to want to get out of bed or move from our couch, never mind attempting anything as adventurous as hiking while on holiday, or playing with the grandkids in the yard. This creates a conflict in our minds, because sightseeing is a wonderful experience, and taking time to engage with our families creates precious memories that can never be replaced. Those wants are sidelined by the fear of experiencing more pain.

What a bargain grandchildren are! I give them my loose change, and they give me a million dollars' worth of pleasure. -Gene Perret

Slowing down with aging doesn't need to take away those things that you love to take part in. **With just 10 minutes a day, you can transform your life back into one full of action and joy.**

Your hobbies and passions don't need to be out of bounds for you because your body is failing you. But, let's be honest, we do put our bodies through a lot by the time we reach our 50s, so perhaps it is time that we give a little back to them. Making the choice today to set yourself up for a healthier future by starting to take care of your muscles and joints now is never going to be a choice that you will regret.

Regular consistent stretching can:

- reduce pain
- improve posture
- improve balance
- improve flexibility
- increase your energy levels
- decrease stress

Learning to reverse your bad habits, loosen stiff joints and strengthen muscles that you forgot you even owned, can all contribute to increasing your confidence to take part in the things that you have been missing. You can take part in an impromptu game of tag with the grandchildren, accept your friend's invitation to explore a new city on a weekend break, get away somewhere quiet with your partner, and enjoy the great outdoors. Whatever it is that makes you feel joy can be regained.

My aim is to help you become more confident on your feet, pain-free, and mobile. In this book, I will explain why aging happens and how it affects us, why you should pre-prepare your exercise space, and the importance of doing warm-ups. The book will also show you why stretching is important and how it can contribute to managing common aches and pains.

In the book, key stretches for all different parts of the body, tailored to many different ability levels, are broken down into easy-to-follow step-by-step instructions, accompanied by illustrations that show you how to do it.

I also cover how you can make the most of additional tools to take your exercise routine to the next level and get yourself to even greater health levels.

Chapter 1:

What Happens as We Age?

For most people, aging is first noticed by us as tiredness, that feeling that your grandkids are a lot harder to keep up with than your kids ever were. For many, deteriorating eyesight is one of the first outwardly noticeable changes in their body, and the percentage of the population requiring corrective lenses dramatically increases past the age of 45.

You might have caught yourself starting to make grunts when you stand up, or try to get out of bed. You also probably are all too aware of simply not feeling as strong or agile as you used to be, and everything just seems to ache all the time, with no rhyme or reason. A lot of people develop regional conditions that can weaken joints and limbs, compounding the effects of aging even further.

There is more to aging, however, than the surface symptoms that you initially notice. The saying that "Age never comes alone" is certainly true; to understand how it affects us, and how in turn, we can combat it, we first need to understand what happens inside our bodies as we enter this stage in our lives.

How Does the Body Age?

Aging isn't just a passage of time; it's a process that all of our bodies go through as a result of our cellular makeup. The cells that all of the bones, and soft tissues of our bodies comprise, are preprogrammed to divide continually, therefore increasing their numbers. There are two main reasons for this; the first is to allow us to grow, and the second is to continually repair bodily structures. This is how we heal ourselves after receiving a cut or bruise, and how we replace cells that we regularly shed, like skin, or hair.

Somatic cells - the non-reproductive cells that are found in all other structures of the body - divide in a process known as mitosis. During this process, the cell divides itself into two by creating a replica of itself (Schermelleh, 2014).

Though the cells created are theoretically identical copies of each other, they actually lose a little of their quality each time they divide. It is a bit like using a photocopier to reproduce a letter template, and then using that template copy to photocopy the next batch, and keeping one of those new copies for the next time you need to print more etc. Each time you make a new copy of your template, the type gets more blurry, and the background becomes more and more shadowy, seemingly from nowhere. Just like how you will experience a reduced ability to read the remaining text on these copies, resulting in the function of the template in the first place becoming lost, the equivalent loss in quality of the cell, translates to a loss in its original function, eventually leading the cell to the point where it is no longer able to divide at all, and it ultimately dies.

The science behind why this happens is called the telomere theory of aging. Scientists studying DNA have identified an area at the end of each chromosome-pairs of DNA that govern how every cell works by storing its genetic code-named the telomere. Some people refer to this as the "junk DNA" because it doesn't do anything to the cell, it doesn't contain any DNA code instructions for the working of it, or dictate how it should grow. However, the telomere does have an important role to play when it comes to cell division, it acts as a handle on the end of the chromosome where the copying process can begin (Fossel, 2017, p.37).

Going back to our photocopier analogy, if your copier were a handheld scanner, the telomere would be the corner of the page that you would have to hold in order to keep it still while you perform the scan. Each time you scan, you lose more detail from that corner because you are covering it with your hand. Eventually, the detail lost in the corner begins to include some of the words that you needed to be able to see on your template. This happens in the cells too; the more times they divide, the more of the telomere handle is lost. Once a great deal of the telomere is gone, the cell can't reproduce anymore without missing out on some of its important DNA information, so mitosis stops.

After cells stop dividing, or their quality becomes low enough to result in a negative effect on the wider structure that it is part of, we start to see signs of aging appear. If we think of cells as the building blocks of our tissues, then it becomes easy to understand how faults in these blocks, or even missing blocks, will result in 'cracks' in the larger structure.

In skin, for example, this manifests as a thinning of the outer layer, and a loss of elasticity. You might notice the skin around your upper arms becoming looser, or an appearance of jowls on your neck. Have you had bruises appear from nowhere, or noticed that a cut on your finger has taken what feels like forever to heal? This is a result of slower healing due to fewer cells dividing too.

Loss of bone density is common as we get older, and especially so in women and people with a uterus, once their hormones start to change around their menopause. You may know about, or even have osteoporosis, or osteoarthritis yourself, both are conditions that result from a reduced rate of cell renewal in our bones, causing weaknesses and leading to an increased risk of fractures.

There are numerous other examples of how the death of cells results in poor performance of bodily structures, but for the purposes of this book, we will only look further into how this manifests ailments in your joints, and soft tissues - muscles, ligaments, and tendons - and how this impacts the way senior bodies move.

Structure of Joints

In order to understand how an ailment becomes a problem for the health of our joints, we first need to understand what happens in a normally functioning joint. Though there are many types of joints found in the human body, they all have a commonly shared purpose, to facilitate the effective meeting point of two or more bones in the skeleton, and to allow for points of movement to originate from them.

The type of joint that is most relevant to our mobility is known as a synovial joint. While some joints are immobile, or even fused, the synovial joints are the ones responsible for creating movement in our limbs. They are found in your shoulders, elbows, wrists, hips, knees, and ankles. They are also found in areas where bones may move alongside each other independently, such as in the hands and feet. These joints can be further classified into one of five types:

- plane joint: where bones have limited movement range and can only slide or twist against each other

- saddle joint: where convex and concave bone surfaces cover each other similar to a rider saddled on a horse. These joints typically only allow for movement in one plane, though the bones may also be able to slide over each other

- hinge joint: where the bones are developed to closely fit one another, and strongly supported by collateral ligaments to prevent movement, dictating that the joint can only move in a single plane

- pivot joint: where one bone forms an axial pivot and an adjoining bone forms a complete ring which will only allow the joint to rotate in place

- ball and socket joint: where the end of one bone forms a ball-like structure, and the adjoining bone features a concave surface across which the ball can move. This joint type is the most mobile, allowing for movement in all planes

No matter the classification shape, synovial joints all share common structural components, even when the movements they create are different in type from one another.

In synovial joints, you will find the following structures:

- articular cartilage
- synovial cavity
- joint capsule
- synovial lining
- ligaments
- tendons
- bursa

Each structure has its own role within these mobile joints; a dysfunction in any one or more of them can result in an unhealthy joint, causing stiffness, pain, or a loss of stability.

Articular cartilage is a tough, fibrous tissue that covers the ends of bones where they meet each other. The tissue is also extremely smooth, creating a functional surface that allows the bones to glide freely over one another, while simultaneously protecting the bones from wearing each other down.

The synovial cavity is the gap between the intersection of two or more bones, and is the area where synovial fluid is found. This fluid is a non-newtonian substance, which allows it to become thicker when put under pressure. It is the part of our joints that cushions all of the other structures, protecting them from the loads that they have to bear, and providing shock absorbency. The synovial cavity is enclosed by the synovial lining, which has a dual function. It produces synovial fluid for the joint, and traps that fluid within the cavity, preventing it from spilling out and being lost when pressure is put on the joint. Bursas are also found in several areas of the body, and can lay between ligaments and bones, or multiple ligaments. They are small cushions of the synovial membrane that contain synovial fluid, and protect other component parts of joints from wear as they move over each other. They aren't found constantly in all synovial joints, but since they are essentially a miniature joint capsule, I have included them here.

The structures covered so far allow for free movement and protection of the joint, however if these were the only components present, a joint would be unstable and have no control applied to the level of movement it is allowed to perform. The skeleton would simply fall apart at the joints. To prevent this, synovial joints have both stabilizing structures - ligaments, and structures that perform the task of intended movements - muscles.

Ligaments are fibrous tissues made of collagen. They consist of thousands of fibers all running parallel to one another, making them especially good at resisting damage from pulling forces. They join bones to other bones and are responsible for limiting the movement of joints, so that your bones will not slide apart from each other. Damaged ligaments will repair by creating scar tissue; although a healed ligament will still add stability to a joint, the new tissue will not be as strong as it was before the injury occurred.

Tendons are also made up of collagen fibers; their function is to connect muscles to bones. They provide an anchor on which a muscle can pull to create the desired movement. There are often several tendons around the same joint, in order to create a number of different possible movement types, over different directions. Injured or damaged tendons reduce the muscle's ability to effectively pull on its connecting bone, and can result in reduced strength when performing their normal functions. As with ligaments, damaged tendons can heal by creating scar tissue, but they will not retain their original level of strength.

Joint Stiffness and Extended Sitting

Joint stiffness increases as we age because our bodies become less able to maintain our soft tissues. We may lose muscle mass, experience tighter and shorter ligaments, or become subject to cartilage loss. We also find it more difficult to keep all of these soft tissues sufficiently hydrated.

The health of our joints is commonly accessed by checking the degree of flexibility that they have. Flexibility is the ability for your joints to move freely through their normal, full range of motion-ROM-, without pain (Bataineh, 2021). There are several different types of joints in our bodies, each that move on different planes, for example: up v down, side to side, or rotational actions. For each joint, a healthy ROM means that you can easily maneuver yourself from its tightest position to its most open position without resistance. The best way to maintain flexibility is to regularly use your muscles to keep them active and prevent over-tightening or reduction in length. It is important to keep your joints moving daily, if you don't use your full ROM regularly, it will decline.

Causes of joint stiffness can include, torn or inflamed cartilage-often seen in rheumatoid arthritis, shortened or stiffened ligaments and tendons which limit ROM, the effect of which is similar to a door closure that is too tight and won't allow you to fully open the door in the first place, or muscle weakness resulting in the joint being unable to sufficiently *close*.

In addition to this, the free movement of our body and joints depends on the fundamental ability for us to be able to maintain a solid center of gravity. Since we have evolved to be bipedal - walk upright on two feet - our skeletons and musculature have also evolved to maintain that upright position with minimal effort. The curvature of the spine, and load-bearing ability of our knees, and ankles, are the most notable of these evolved traits. It could be argued that this is an example of great natural engineering making the most of our upright forms. I would agree; however, this specialization then becomes a problem when we spend extended amounts of time sitting.

Humans are not 'designed' to be sitting at a desk for multiple hours every day, sitting in a car commuting long distances, or even slouching on a couch with the TV every evening after dinner. Sitting changes our center of gravity; it alters the way our skeleton has to hold the weight of our own bodies, and puts pressure on joints in a different way than how they evolved to handle it.

As well as putting increased pressure on your joints, it can lead to tightened hip flexors and hamstring muscles, which in turn makes it more difficult to walk. These changes reduce the length of your strides and can also cause you to lean forward, both of which increase the danger of a trip or fall, on top of increasing the amount of effort that you need to put into getting around. You may have noticed this in yourself or other people who have the appearance of a frontward curved spine and lowered head, and who characteristically shuffle their feet instead of taking full strides.

There are other dangers of sitting for long periods of time, besides mobility problems too. Studies have indicated that extended sitting can lead to weight gain, diabetes, heart disease, varicose veins or thrombosis, digestive problems, and depressed mood (Department of Health, State Government of Victoria, Australia, 2018).

Importance of Movement

Joint stiffness, though generally initially caused by aging tissue, or injury, will become a destructive cycle if not addressed. What I mean by this is: when you have a stiff joint, it can be sore enough to make you unwilling to move it around, nobody wants to cause themselves pain if they can help it. In turn, this makes the condition worse, and it will become even more painful. This is why you may notice your joints feel stiffer when you wake up than at night, and they gradually ease through the day, after you start to move around.

There are of course, also emotional well-being reasons why you will want to keep the ability to move without pain or stiffness. You might have grandchildren you desperately want to be able to look after safely, want to be able to continue working, or even just want to keep your independence by being able to run errands and do housework unaided. Not to mention that chronically occurring pain can cause a depressed mood or anxiety. Being free to move around without pain gives us confidence and self-esteem boosts, but can also lead to a reduction in stress, and better sleep.

The Arthritis and Rheumatism Associates, P.C. (Bowen, 2022), explains that our bodies operate on the principle of move it or lose it, but that the effects of aging can be slowed, and sometimes reversed by keeping active.

There are other physical benefits to making an effort to reduce the amount of time we are sedentary during the day too. You can improve the condition of your bones and muscles, becoming stronger and feeling less tired. People who are more active after 65 can experience a longer life expectancy, reduce the likelihood of trips and falls, and reduce their risk of developing chronic diseases. Additionally, keeping your body healthy can help to keep your medical costs down.

Benefits of Stretching

As you have seen, there are a ton of reasons why you might want to get the benefits of keeping active, but why does stretching in particular help you to achieve that? Regular stretching routines can lengthen ligaments and tendons, regain muscle mass and strength, reduce pain and inflammation, and improve overall flexibility. In a nutshell, it improves our ability to perform the full ROM of all our joints, which can lead to a number of knock-on benefits.

If falls, in particular, are a worrisome thought for you, you'll be reassured to know that stretching also improves posture, which improves your ability to balance effectively and helps us to be more steady on our feet. Becoming more flexible, and gaining confidence to move around safely, will ultimately allow you to be more active in all other areas of your life, improve your mood, and reduce the risk of trips or falls.

If you suffer from lower limb problems such as peripheral artery disease, or poor circulation in relation to diabetes, you might also find it reassuring that studies have indicated regular stretching increases blood flow to the muscles (Geriatric Medicine Journal, 2018). Increased health of the lower limbs as a result of improved blood supply can go on to improve mobility for those who may have previously been limited by pain or associated foot conditions. It also ensures that there is a readily available source of oxygen for your muscles to use during movement, reducing soreness after activity.

A regular and long-term stretching routine can help to reduce pain by strengthening joints and restoring lost ROM. Taking the time out of our busy lives to perform stretching plans will give us a much-needed break from the 'daily grind', that we ordinarily may not prioritize for ourselves. It provides us with a few minutes every day where we can be calm, center ourselves on the task at hand,

and gain some relaxation, whilst performing a mild activity to improve our physical health. Since stretching is a gentle and slow practice, some people even choose to practice mindfulness techniques alongside it.

Chapter 2:

What Is Stretching?

Stretching, as it relates to physical health and fitness, is the process of placing particular parts of the body into a position that will lengthen, or elongate, the muscles and associated soft tissues. Upon undertaking a regular stretching program a number of changes begin to occur within the body and specifically within the muscles themselves. Other tissues that begin to adapt to the stretching process include the fascia, tendons, ligaments, skin and scar tissue. -
Walker, 2021

Types of Stretch

Stretches generally fit into one of two type groupings: static stretches, and dynamic stretches. This means that stretches are intended to be done either by relaxing into a still pose, or whilst working the muscles through the ROM for a joint. Each type has its own advantages and disadvantages.

Static Stretching Types

The static stretching group of activity can be further broken down into five more sub-categories: traditional static, assisted or passive, active, isometric, and proprioceptive neuromuscular facilitation-PNF. That last one is a bit of a mouthful, but don't worry about remembering the full term; PNF is essentially a type of stretch where contracted muscles are guided through their range of motion with the assistance of a trainer or other health care professional.

I want you to be able to take control of your own health improvement. For this reason, I won't be teaching you PNF stretching in this book. Instead, I will cover the passive, static, and isometric stretch types from this grouping of stretches.

Dynamic Stretching Types

Dynamic stretching, as it suggests, is a more dynamic way of applying a stretch. It focuses on the daily function of your joints, and applies the stretch to your soft tissue as you move it through the ROM, rather than in a single position. This type grouping includes: traditional dynamic, ballistic, active isolated stretching, and resistance or loaded stretching. From this group, you will learn traditional dynamic activities in this book.

Stretching Sub-types Featured in This Book

To bring that all together, this book will take you through four subtypes of stretches in total: static, passive, isometric, and dynamic. The reasoning behind this choice is all about their function, and how they affect your joints' functioning too. The subtypes included are easier to perform, can be done alone, and are the best types to use for targeting the desired goals of improving posture and reducing joint pain so that you can feel confident to remain active safely.

Static stretching is the type of activity that most people think of when they imagine a stretching program. Muscle groups are targeted by adopting specific postures intended to target desired muscle groups and holding that pose until the muscles are given time to relax into that position, and lengthen. This stretch can be used easily for rehabilitation of injury as it doesn't put any strain or burden on the joint while the muscles stretch.

Passive stretches are very similar to static poses; however, the key difference is that during a passive stretch, the person remains relaxed and will use an external aid to push or pull the muscles into their furthest point of ROM. The external aid could be someone helping you if you have a willing family member that you trust to respect your limits. Tools such as therapy bands are a great alternative to enlisting help; for some stretches of the lower body; you can use your hands to assist the lower joints too. The main benefit of passive stretching is that it can help lengthen muscles without requiring the muscle to do the active work of getting into that position before the benefits can be achieved. In other words, if you have lost strength in some muscle groups, you can still reach the required stretch for that area, even if you are normally unable to maneuver into that position using the action of that muscle group alone.

Isometric stretches can put more pressure on a joint than static or passive do, and so should be done less frequently. However, the trade-off is that this particular type of stretch specifically targets your ability to strengthen joints by activating the muscle groups around them. While passive and static target a lengthening of your muscles to be able to perform full ROM, isometric utilizes tensing muscle groups in a stable stretch pose to build strength.

Lastly, we have dynamic stretching. This kind of stretch adds a level of complexity by working the muscle groups through the whole ROM. It builds from isometric stretching to ensure that the strength you gain from activating the muscles can be functionally used in the whole range, in your daily routines. This means that you will be able to actively move your joints through their ROM during activity safely, not only when you are standing or sitting still. This stretch is key to helping you keep on top of all the things you like to do daily. It focuses on ensuring that you can perform all the motions that you need in order to live your life without restriction.

It aims for you to be able to dress comfortably and unaided, brush your hair or teeth alone, use your stairs confidently, and work through other chores or errands, retaining your independence.

What Makes It a Good Stretch?

To gain the best results from your stretches you need to ensure that you are using proper form every time you undertake them. Stretches performed without due care to the technique can be harmful, and may even exacerbate pain, or cause, injury. No individual stretch is inherently 'bad' in itself, but all of them have the potential to become damaging, if not done correctly. This is why you will frequently see personal trainers, or coaches, correcting the form of their clients.

To avoid doing it 'badly,' we, by definition, would need to aim for a 'good' stretch, or technique in order to prevent potential damage from occurring.

How do you know if it is a 'good' one or not? Here are some tips on how to ensure you are doing everything you can to perform your stretching routines safely. Be sure to warm-up prior to stretching; a light jog on the spot or a few laps of your couch is a fine place to start if you have limited mobility, or low fitness levels and are just starting out. The next step is to have the confidence to listen to your body; you know if something doesn't feel right, and you know where your limits are. Don't push yourself too hard; forcing your joints into a stretch can cause injury and set you back in your progress. Stretching can be uncomfortable but should never be painful, if you experience pain, ease back, and consider an alternative until you are able to try again in the future. Remember, you should only be stretching until you feel tension on the muscle, it should be enjoyable and relaxing, don't push your stretch past the point of resistance and into pain.

Ensure that you move into your stretches slowly, and avoid bouncing your joints as this can be harmful. It can push you into your areas of pain before you have a chance to recognize that you are approaching your limit. A bounce during stretching would also push your stretch out of the static grouping and into ballistic stretching.

Common Stumbling Blocks

Don't forget to continue breathing during the entirety of your stretching routine. It may sound odd, but it's a common mistake for beginners to hold their breath. This makes their muscles tense and lowers the effectiveness of the stretch by reducing the range of stretch that can be achieved. It also makes it more difficult to perform the stretch. Breathe slowly and calmly, fill your whole chest, and practice belly breathing - as much as you are able; this may be dependent on any lung conditions you might have; as before, listen to your body. If you have a chest condition that you know limits your breathing, you might also want to consider building longer breaks into your routine between different stretches.

When you have medical conditions that may restrict your ability to perform some stretches, you shouldn't allow it to prevent you from taking part altogether. There are ways to adapt your stretches to make them more appropriate and comfortable for you. For example, if you experience poor balance, you can hold onto the back of a chair, or your kitchen counters, to support you in standing stretches. You can stick to sitting in a chair when stretching if you get tired easily when standing for an extended time. If you have an injury, avoid stretching the area for at least 72 hours following the occurrence. For 10 to 14 days afterward you can do some light stretches, but avoid anything more intensive than static stretches until after the second week. It can take 12 weeks for a soft tissue injury to heal, so be mindful of your recovery progress while stretching, and don't ramp things up too quickly. If you feel that you overdid it in one session, there is no shame in paring back your next few sessions. Allowing time and care to properly heal injuries will always be more important than pushing yourself to stick to your old levels of activity.

Specific injury aside, it's important to remember that it took months, or even years for your joints to stiffen and muscles to become shortened. You can't reverse this deterioration overnight, so don't get discouraged if you don't immediately see results. A consistent effort to stretch daily will result in gradual, sustained, improvements. However, it doesn't take hours and hours every day to get the benefits of stretching. All you need is to dedicate 10 minutes a day; it is really a question of quality over quantity when it comes to your daily routine.

Stretches should be held for between 30 to 60 seconds; this gives the muscles a chance to relax into the new stretched position that we want them to adapt to. Each stretch should also be repeated two to three times. Don't panic about fitting three lots of 60-second stretches across your whole body into one 10-minute daily routine; stretching everything at once isn't necessary. If you aren't experiencing pain normally, or a joint is perfectly capable of moving through its whole ROM without issue, then you don't need to stretch it, and you can focus instead on your personal problem areas first.

Prepare for Success

I have no doubt that you have heard the phrase "dressing for success." This applies to exercise as much as it does in any other situation. Choose clothes that will allow you to perform your stretches without being restricted by the material. Be cautious, though, not to choose anything too baggy; a simple mistake of trapping some of the material under the foot can result in a nasty fall. A key checklist for choosing your clothes should also include: breathable materials, either cotton or specialized sportswear, and looking for a level of stretch that allows you to freely move.

You're going to need to select appropriate footwear too. Opt for athletic shoes that are flat-soled to avoid slipping on smooth floors. If you are stretching at home you may choose to complete your stretches barefoot instead, this avoids your ankle ROM being restricted by any shoes you have on and can help you to relax.

Once your clothes are prepared, you will want to ensure you have a safe space to work in. Be sure there isn't clutter in your exercise area, and be sure to put any pets outside the room for the duration so that they won't get underfoot while you are stretching.

Gather a blanket or exercise mat to improve comfort when you are working through floor stretches. Be sure whatever you choose to use has a good grip on the floor and won't slide around while you are stretching. It also needs to be stable; avoid using thick duvets or soft comforters as they can be difficult to balance on. If you choose to purchase an exercise mat, look for something made of either rubber or jute. As stretching isn't high impact, a 0.1" yoga mat would work perfectly well; however, if you have particularly hard floors, you may be more comfortable using a full exercise mat which should be at least 0.5" thick. In terms of size, you're going to want a mat that is at least 6" longer than you are tall; this is to ensure you have sufficient cover to perform stretches lying down in comfort. You won't want to be able to feel the edge of the mat underneath you; at best, it can be distracting, and at worst, it might be painful.

For chair exercises, you need to choose a chair that is secure and without any damage. Look for something with a solid seat, such as a dining chair. Avoid using a couch as it can lead to restricted movement, doesn't support you, and can encourage slouching.

Get yourself a towel so that you can wipe away any sweat during your routine and stay comfortable. Avoid eating right before stretching, but do drink water and bring an extra bottle to your stretching area too. You will be losing water through your sweat, and your breathing while you exercise, which will need to be replaced. Hydration is often forgotten about when stretching, even though most people would be able to tell you that it is key to any other type of exercise. Muscles use water as well as oxygen as fuel when they work out; remembering to drink throughout your session will reduce tiredness and the risk of cramps. Becoming dehydrated during exercise can cause drowsiness, and increase your core temperature, making your exercise harder to perform.

When and Where to Stretch

When to Stretch

You'll probably remember being told to stretch before and after workouts, but I don't recommend doing it afterward. It is worth noting that stretches can be performed in isolation from any other type of workout warm-ups; being the exception, you should always warm up. In fact, stretching in the morning before getting on with the rest of your day can help reduce stiffness and get you moving faster, dispelling any discomfort from the night before and giving you an energy boost. Stretching before bedtime can also be beneficial for different reasons; it relieves tension built up throughout the day, relaxing your muscles, and your mind too, helping you get a better night's sleep.

If you work behind a desk, or find yourself spending a lot of time on the couch, it is also recommended to take regular stretching breaks. This can alleviate tension, improve mood, and increase blood flow and digestion. If possible, getting up to perform gentle stretches after every hour can make a big impact on your mood and ability to focus.

Where to Stretch

Since stretching doesn't require a lot of equipment, you can do it almost anywhere. Though, there are a few things to take into consideration that can make your experience more comfortable. Try to choose a temperature-controlled environment to keep you warm. Besides being generally unpleasant, being cold when you stretch can lead to injury. It's a good idea to choose places where you can relax. Some people find that getting some calming music to listen to while they stretch helps them to find relaxation.

Chapter 3:

Warming Up

Why Should You Warm Up?

Clinical studies suggest that warming up before exercise increases the effectiveness of your workout (Fradkin et al., 2010). A successful warm-up routine will gently take your body from a state of rest to one primed for activity. Aerobically targeted warm ups in particular, have been credited for increasing blood flow, and the availability of oxygen to your muscles, reducing muscle tension.

Other benefits of warming up include: a reduced risk of injury, reduced chance of muscle cramps during exercise, and reduced soreness afterward. There is also the added bonus that a well-rounded warm-up will help you to prepare mentally for your upcoming workout. It gives you time to remember the goals that you have for your exercises, and an opportunity to relax into your routine, increasing the chances of you continuing it in the long term.

The aim of your warm-up is to maintain a slow and steady pace. You want to get your blood pumping and feel ready to stretch safely; you don't want to wear yourself out with it, or perform anything that may force your muscles into a stretch before you are ready.

Warms Ups I Recommend

I have included for you below a program of three warm-up exercises that I recommend you do before every stretching session. Each of these exercises should be conducted for 40 seconds, followed by a 20-second break, and then repeated once more each. Your total warm-up should take approximately five minutes and follow the pattern listed below:

1. marches (40s), then rest (20s)

2. marches (40s), then rest (20s)

3. air boxing (40s), then rest (20s)

4. air boxing (40s), then rest (20s)

5. step back and reach (40s), then rest (20s)

6. step back and reach (40s), then rest (20s)

Be sure to keep taking sips of water during your rests in order to stay hydrated throughout the warm-up.

If you have pre-existing injuries, or conditions, that you feel will stop you from being able to perform the warm-ups recommended, you can substitute them for other techniques to suit your ability level. Walking, running, or spinning are all great substitutes. If you choose to use one of these other methods, be sure to do them for at least five minutes. The goal is still to increase your body temperature, and get blood pumping to your muscles before stretching.

Marches

Marching on the spot will provide a warm-up to your hip flexor muscles, and engage your ankles, and your core. As you march and switch from one foot to another, your center of gravity will constantly change, giving your body an opportunity to practice your ability to balance effectively too. It is the best place to start in order to get your blood pumping, and raise your temperature.

Step by step:

1. stand with your feet hip-width apart

2. raise your left leg, bending at the knee as you bring it up to your hip

3. bend your elbows and raise your right arm in time with your left leg, until your upper arm is shoulder height and parallel to the floor

4. simultaneously lower your left leg and right arm

5. switch sides, raising your right leg with your left arm

6. continue to alternate so that you are marching on the spot

To get the best results from your marches, aim to bring your knees up as high as possible without pushing yourself into discomfort. Pump your arms up and down in time with your steps, ensuring to keep your elbows bent, but don't clench your fists. Keep marching for 40 seconds, take your 20-seconds break, and repeat the whole process before moving on to the next warm-up.

If you cannot perform marches while standing, it can be substituted for leg lifts in a chair. Sit straight in your chair with your feet hip-width apart and lift your knees as far as is comfortable. Alternate your knee lifts and pump your arms to help raise your heart rate.

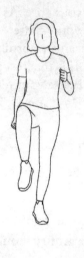

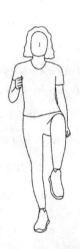

Air Boxing

Air boxing will warm up your shoulders, arms and core. Since you will be extending your arms away from your body, it also gives you an opportunity to practice shifting your center of gravity to compensate for the weight of your arm being taken away from your center.

Step by step:

1. stand with one leg in front of the other and a slight bend to your knees

2. hold your arms in front of your chest, bent at the elbows and with a loose fist

3. slowly extend your left arm out, punching forward

4. return your left arm to its original position in front of your chest

5. slowly extend your right arm out, punching forward

6. return your right arm to its original position in front of your chest

7. repeat, continuing to alternate your arms, for 40 seconds

For your starting stance, you can put forward whichever foot is the most comfortable for you, and will make you feel most confident about standing stably. Keep your arms at shoulder height as you extend them and bring them back. Aim to fully extend and retract your arms before switching sides to avoid the tendency of swinging your body from side to side.

Keep air boxing for 40 seconds, and remember to take your 20-second break before repeating. Then take another 20-second rest and move on to the next warm-up.

If you are unable to stand comfortably to perform air boxing, you can make use of a chair to support you. Sit straight in your chair, with your feet flat on the floor, and box the air with your arms. Be sure not to slouch, as this will decrease your ability to properly extend and retract your arms.

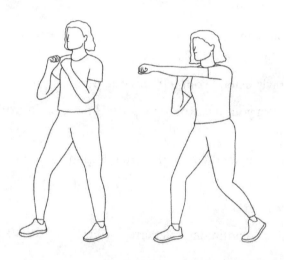

Step Back and Reach

The step back and reach will warm up your back, core, arms, and legs. It helps to pump blood around your whole body as well as improve your balance. It also opens your ribcage, encouraging you to take deeper breaths, and increasing your oxygen intake.

Step by step:

1. start with your legs shoulder-width apart and a slight bend in your knees

2. step back with one foot as far as is comfortable for you

3. raise your arms into the air, reaching as far up to the sky as you can

4. lower your arms and return your feet to the starting position

5. then step back using your opposite leg, repeating the reach with your arms

6. return to the center and repeat for 40 seconds, continuing to alternate from one leg to the other

The aim is to feel a slight stretch from your calves and thighs, up though your spine each time that you reach up. If you have particularly tight hamstrings or calves, this may feel very uncomfortable, if it hurts, you can lower the intensity by bending the knee of the leg that you step back onto or reducing the length of your stride.

Keep alternating the side that you step back onto for 40 seconds, then be sure to take your 20 seconds rest before you repeat the process. Afterwards, take another 20 seconds break before moving on to your stretching.

If you find this too difficult, you can lower the difficulty by performing a reach on a chair. Sit straight in your chair with your feet flat on the floor. Raise both hands over your head and stretch upwards as far as you can. Lower your arms, and repeat.

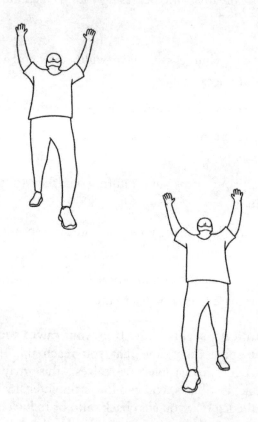

Chapter 4:

Upper Body Chair Exercises

Side Neck Hold

Muscles Targeted: sternocleidomastoid, scalene, longissimus capitis, splenius capitis, semispinalis capitis, and upper trapezius.

Step by step:

1. sit straight in your chair with your feet flat on the floor

2. breathe in, and breathe out as you tilt your head to the left

3. lift your left arm up over your head, grasping your head with your palm across the crown and your fingers pointing towards your right ear

4. gently pull your head downward to your shoulder

5. hold for 30-60 seconds

6. repeat on the opposite side

The action you are looking for is to bring your ear towards your shoulder, breathe out as you settle into the pose, and remember not to hold your breath once you are in position. Avoid applying excessive force, and remember to pull back, if you experience any pain. Practice keeping a straight back posture while you do this, and try not to let your head dip forwards, especially if you normally spend a lot of time looking at screens.

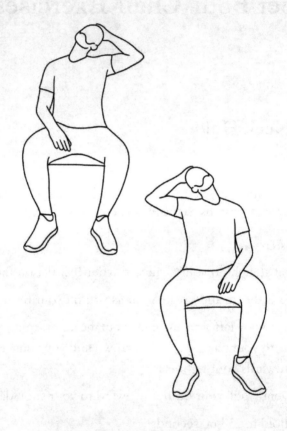

Frontal Shoulder Stretch

Muscles targeted: triceps, posterior deltoid, trapezius group, teres group, rhomboid and latissimus dorsi.

Step by step:

1. sit straight in your chair with your feet flat on the floor.

2. breathe in as you raise your left arm above your head.

3. keep your arm straight so that it rests against your left ear.

4. use your right hand to grasp your left elbow.

5. breath out, and gently pull your left arm backward past your ear, using your right arm to control the motion.

6. hold this position for 30-60 seconds.

7. gently release and lower your arms, then repeat on the opposite side.

Remember to avoid holding your breath while you stretch. It is a common mistake to suck in air as you pull your arm back, and hold onto it until you release your arms. Doing this encourages you to drop your arms too quickly, tenses the muscles in the chest, and reduces the stretch at the arm, as well as reduces oxygen in the blood flow. Avoid dipping your head forward while you perform this stretch; the aim is to pull your arm back and open up the chest, not stretch the back of the neck.

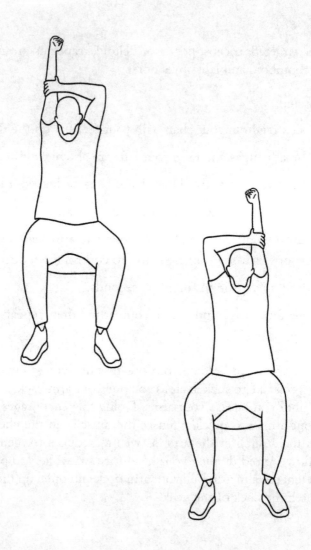

Lateral Shoulder Stretch

Muscles targeted: mid and posterior deltoid, triceps, teres group, latissimus dorsi, and serratus anterior.

Step by step:

1. sit straight in your chair with your feet flat on the floor
2. lift your left arm up to shoulder height and then cross it in front of your chest with your thumb pointing downwards
3. bend your right arm at the elbow and cross your right forearm in front of your left arm
4. use your right arm like a 'hook' to gently pull your left arm into your chest and across to the right
5. breath out and relax into the position as you pull
6. hold this position for 30-60 seconds
7. gently release your arms and repeat on the opposite side

Avoid holding your breath or shrugging your shoulders upwards as you perform this stretch. You shouldn't be able to feel your arm pressing against your neck. Aim to keep your torso facing forwards; while it is natural for your shoulder to round the side of your chest a little during this stretch, you should avoid twisting your body. This is a beginner mistake that some people mistake for gaining a deeper stretch of the shoulder.

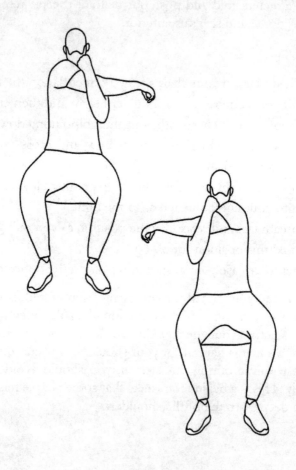

Trunk Rotations

Muscles targeted: rectus abdominis, internal and external oblique.

Step by step:

1. sit straight in your chair with your feet flat on the floor
2. lift your left arm over the back of your chair and grip the top with your hand
3. reach your right arm across the front of your body to grip the left side of your chair
4. slowly breathe out as you twist your torso to the left as far as is comfortable for you
5. slowly turn back to center
6. place your right arm over the back of your chair
7. reach your left arm across the front of your body to grip the right side of the chair
8. slowly breathe out as you twist your torso to the right
9. repeat, alternating sides 5-8 times in each direction

The action you are aiming for her, is to end looking over the back of your chair, using your hands to support you as you do. Not everyone will be able to twist the full way around, and this is normal, especially if you are at the beginning of your stretching journey. Though it is natural for your hips to turn slightly as you do this stretch, avoid lifting them up off the chair.

If you find this stretch too difficult, you can adapt it by crossing your arms in front of your chest, with your palms on the front of your shoulders, and turning your upper torso by 90 degrees in each direction. A possible substitute for this stretch could also be to use the lying T-twist from chapter eight: upper body floor stretches, instead.

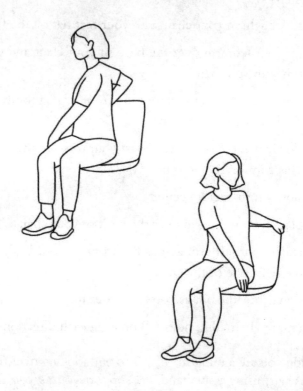

Overhead Stretch

Muscles targeted: pectoralis major and minor.

Step by step:

1. sit straight in your chair facing forward, with your feet flat on the floor
2. breathe in as you raise both of your arms high above your head
3. pull your shoulder blades together to open your chest
4. look up to the ceiling as you do this
5. breathe out as you lower your hands back down
6. repeat 5-8 times

Be sure to move slowly through the whole sequence, take a few seconds to breathe and recenter yourself each time you lower your arms if you are finding it difficult. Avoid letting your arms rotate outwards, as this will cause your shoulders to drop and reduce the number of muscles targeted by the stretch. If you feel like you are able to challenge yourself, you can increase the intensity of this stretch by aiming to push your arms back past the line of your ears slightly once they are above your head. If you choose to do this, avoid allowing the weight of your arms to pull your back into a backward bend.

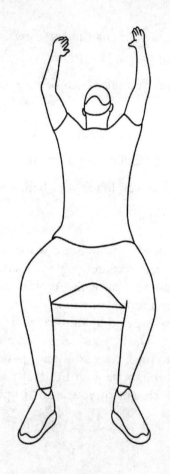

Crescent Moon

Muscles targeted: latissimus dorsi, serratus anterior, and rhomboid.

Step by step:

1. sit straight in your chair with your feet flat on the floor

2. clasp your hands together and raise your arms high over your head

3. breathe out as you lean your upper body over to the left

4. breathe in and straighten your torso, bringing your hands back to the center above your head

5. breathe out again as you lean over to the right

6. repeat this 5-8 times in each direction

The goal is to create a crescent moon, or 'c' shape, with your torso.

If you find it too difficult to hold your hands above your head for the entire time, you can return them to your lap each time you straighten your torso and take a couple of seconds to rest before stretching alternate sides. Should that adaptation not be enough to help reduce the difficulty of this stretch for you, you can leave your arms in your lap while bending to the side, still aiming to achieve a 'c' shape with your torso.

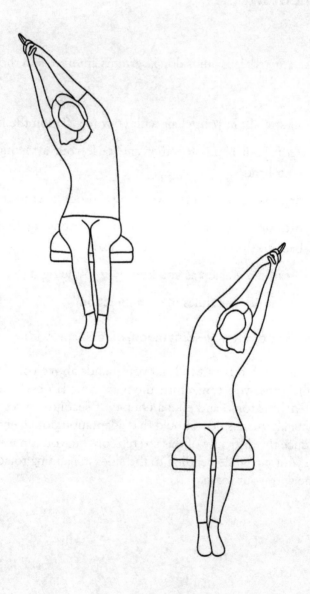

Chapter 5:

Lower Body Chair Exercises

Glute Stretch

Muscles targeted: Gluteus group, piriformis, gemellus group, obturator group, and to a lesser extent the erector spinae.

Step by step:

1. sit straight in the chair facing forward

2. with your knees bent at 90 degrees, lift your left leg and place your ankle on top of your right thigh

3. support your left knee and ankle with your hands and lean forwards.

4. bring your torso over your knees

5. relax into the position and hold it for 30-60 seconds

6. sit up straight and return your left foot to the floor

7. repeat with the opposite leg

Avoid pushing your knee downwards as you lean forwards as this has the potential to cause injury to the knee joint, it will also reduce the effectiveness of the pose. If you feel able to do a deeper stretch, you can take a deep breath and push further forwards as you breathe out. You can also cross the top leg further over the bottom supporting leg; this reduces the forward angle at the hip and intensifies the stretch. Alternatively, if you find this stretch too uncomfortable, you can adapt it to lessen the stretch by reducing the extent to which you lean forward.

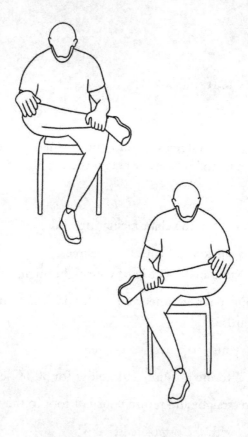

Hamstring Stretch

Muscles targeted: hamstrings, gluteus maximus, gastrocnemius, soleus, and erector spinae.

Step by step:

1. sit on your chair facing forwards

2. stretch both of your legs out in front of you

3. step each foot out to the side so that your feet are a little further apart than the width of your chair

4. place your palms on top of your thighs

5. lean forwards, running your hands down your legs towards your feet as you do

6. breathe out and relax into this position, hold for 30-60 seconds

The aim is to keep your knees straight and hold your ankles with each hand. You may need to shuffle forwards on your chair to be able to do this. Be sure that you slowly return to a sitting position at the end of your stretch. Sitting up too quickly can cause you to become lightheaded. Avoid overextending your knees by transferring your weight onto your legs through your elbows.

If you find this too difficult, you can adapt the stretch by adding a slight bend to your knees, or reducing how far forward you lean into it.

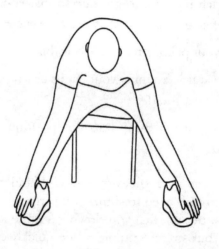

Knee Extensions

Muscles targeted: hamstrings, gastrocnemius, soleus, and tibialis posterior.

Step by step:

1. sit straight in your chair with both feet flat on the floor

2. raise your left leg off the seat slightly, just enough to give your foot free clearance from the floor

3. straighten your left leg in front of you, raising it to hip height

4. bend your left knee to lower your leg back down

5. repeat this movement ten times for the left leg

6. place your left foot back on the floor

7. raise your right leg off the seat

8. straighten your right leg in front of you as you did with your left leg

9. bend your right leg at the knee as you lower it

10. repeat ten times for the right leg

Aim to keep your ankles bent at 90 degrees to your shin; this will improve the stretch in your calves. Remember to perform the movements slowly and maintain even breathing throughout. Avoid leaning your torso forwards, as this will transfer the stretch away from your calves and into your hips.

If this is too difficult for you, or you experience pain in your calves or the sole of your foot, you can adapt the stretch by allowing your toes to point forwards instead of maintaining a 90-degree ankle joint.

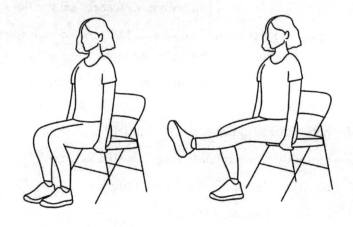

Hip Opener

Muscles targeted: gracilis, hip adductor group, mid-sartorius, and to a lesser extent the gluteus group.

Step by step:

1. sit straight in your chair with your feet flat on the floor

2. keep your knees bent and step your feet out to the sides of your chair, as far as is comfortable for you

3. clasp your hands together and bend your arms.

4. lean forwards and place your elbows to the inside of your legs, just above your knees

5. use your arms to press your knees apart from each other

6. hold this pressure for 30-60 seconds

Aim to keep applying gentle pressure, through your elbows, for the full length of the stretch. If you feel able to push yourself a little further, you can sit further forward on your chair, and tuck your heels against the front chair legs before leaning forward. This is another stretch where you should be careful to not return to an upright position too quickly, to avoid the onset of dizziness.

If you are finding this stretch too difficult, you can decrease the intensity by starting with your elbows closer to your knees, though you should take care to avoid placing them directly on the knee joint.

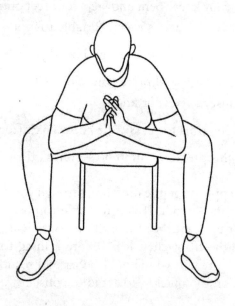

Calf Stretch

For this stretch, you will require an exercise band. If you don't own one, you can substitute with a belt or tie, as long as it is long enough to reach from your feet to your mid-thigh twice. However, it is worth investing in an exercise band due to the gentle resistance they offer, along with the ability to push a stretch further once in place. It is also a very versatile, and relatively inexpensive, piece of equipment that you can make use of in other stretches too.

Muscles targeted: soleus, gastrocnemius, tibialis posterior, flexor digitorum longus, and flexor hallucis longus.

Step by step:

1. sit straight in your chair facing forwards
2. take one end of your exercise band in each hand, forming a loop of material
3. raise your left leg and place your foot into the loop that you created
4. straighten your left leg out in front of you, keeping gentle tension on the band with your hands
5. point your toes to the ceiling
6. pull gently on the band to bring your toes towards you
7. hold this position for 30-60 seconds
8. release the tension on the band carefully before lowering your left leg
9. repeat with the opposite leg

For the greatest benefit, try to keep your ankle at an angle of at least 90 degrees. Avoid yanking on or excessively tugging the exercise band; doing so can overextend the knee and cause injury. This stretch will feel particularly uncomfortable if you are used to spending a lot of time on your feet, especially standing still. Remember to breathe steadily throughout, and avoid allowing your leg to rotate outwards or spread to the side when you apply pressure to the exercise band. If you find it too difficult you can reduce the intensity by adding a slight bend to your knees.

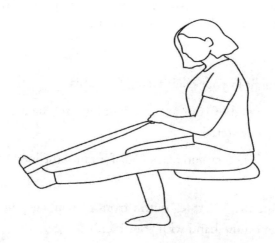

Chapter 6:

Upper Body Wall Stretches

Standing Chest Stretch

Muscles targeted: pectoralis group, serratus anterior, and anterior deltoid.

Step by step:

1. stand facing a wall with your feet hip-width apart

2. raise your left arm out to the side until it reaches shoulder height

3. bend your arm at the elbow, forming a 90-degree angle with your fingers pointing towards the ceiling

4. rest your forearm flat against the wall

5. cross your left foot in front of your right and use the step to rotate your lower body away from the wall

6. keep your left arm flat against the wall and adjust your left foot position for comfort

7. hold for 30-60 seconds

8. turn your torso back to face the wall and lower your arm

9. repeat with the opposite arm

The further you manage to step away from the wall, increasing your torso twist, the deeper this stretch will be. However, be mindful of how your back feels; if the twist causes pain in your back or along the side of your torso, you should reduce the size of the stride that you take when you step around.

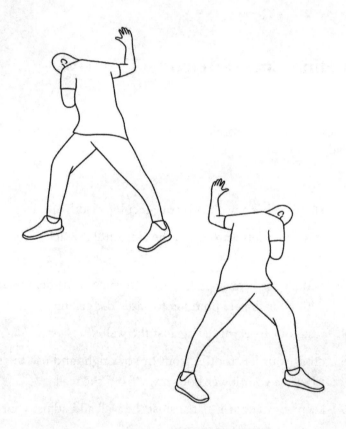

Standing Forearm/Wrist Stretch

Muscles targeted: flexor carpi radialis, flexor carpi ulnaris, flexor digitorum superficialis, and flexor pollicis longus.

Step by step:

1. stand arm's length away from the wall with your feet hip width apart

2. raise your left arm to shoulder height in front of you, keeping your elbow straight

3. bend your wrist to form a 90-degree angle, with your fingers pointing to the ceiling and your palm facing forwards

4. place your fingertips against the wall

5. gently lean forwards into the wall, allowing your wrist to bend further, as far as you are comfortable

6. hold this position for 30-60 seconds

7. stop leaning first, and then allow your arm to come back to your side

8. repeat with the opposite arm

The aim of this stretch is to have the wall assist you in stretching your wrist. You want to avoid forcing your hand back by leaning in too hard, or standing too far away from the wall at the start. Avoid letting your arm rotate either outwards, or inwards, and remember to breathe steadily throughout.

If you are having difficulty performing this stretch, stand closer to the wall and slide your hand up above shoulder height. The higher your reach your arm the easier it will become. You can work on reducing the height of your hand bit by bit in future sessions.

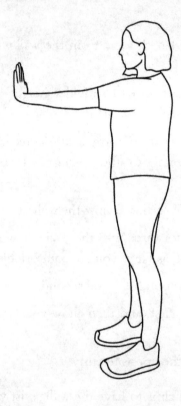

Standing Reverse Forearm/Wrist Stretch

Muscles targeted: flexor digitorum superficialis, flexor carpi ulnaris, flexor carpi radialis, pollicis longus, palmaris longus, pronator teres, brachioradialis, brachialis, and biceps brachii.

Step by step:

1. stand arm's length away from the wall with your feet hip-width apart

2. raise your left arm to shoulder height in front of you, keeping your elbow straight

3. bend your wrist for a 90-degree, with your fingers pointing to the floor and your palm facing forwards

4. place your fingertips against the wall

5. gently lean forwards into the wall, allowing your wrist to bend further and your elbow to straighten as far as you are comfortable

6. hold this position for 30-60 seconds

7. stop leaning first, and then allow your arm to come back to your side

8. repeat with the opposite arm

Aim to keep your whole palm touching the wall. If you work at a desk or spend long periods of time operating machines where your elbows are bent, you may find this particularly uncomfortable at your inner elbow. If this becomes painful at all, then pull back.

If you find this stretch too difficult, you can start with your fingers pointing towards the ceiling, and in increments of approximately 10 degrees, rotate your hand around, away from your body, turning your fingers towards the floor until you feel that you have found your limit. Move back one increment and use that position to hold your stretch for 30-60 seconds. Once this becomes comfortable for you, you can add another increment in your next session and keep progressing until you're able to point your fingers downwards.

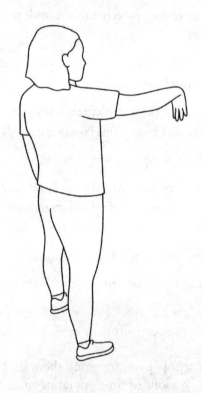

Side Lat Stretch

Muscles targeted: latissimus dorsi, oblique group, rotators, and to a lesser extent, the quadratus lumborum and multifidus.

Step by step:

1. stand arm's length away from the wall, with your left side facing the wall, and feet hip-width apart

2. reach your left arm up until your hand is approximately head height

3. with your fingers pointing to the ceiling, place your palm against the wall

4. lean sideways towards the wall

5. step your left leg forwards, bending the knee slightly to increase the stretch.

6. hold this position for 30-60 seconds

7. gently return to standing upright

8. repeat with your right arm while facing the opposite direction

It is normal for your hips to move away from the wall as you do this; you may want to adjust your footing before holding the stretch to be sure that you have a solid stance.

If you feel you can increase the intensity, you can step further away from the wall to deepen the curve of your torso. Avoid holding your breath during this stretch, as it will contract the muscles we are targeting and reduce the effectiveness of the pose.

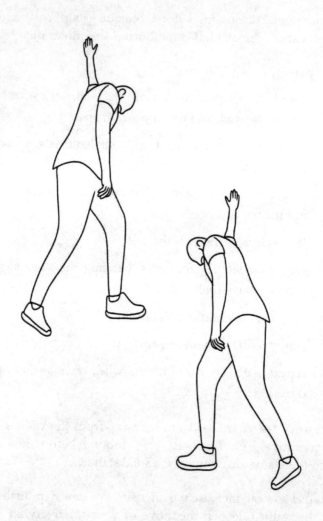

Standing Downward Dog

Muscles targeted: iliocostalis lumborum, multifidus, interspinales, latissimus dorsi, and spinalis thoracis.

Step by step:

1. stand facing the wall with your feet hip-width apart

2. raise both arms to shoulder height

3. with your elbows straight, place your palms against the wall with your fingers pointing to the ceiling

4. step backward away from the wall and lean downwards, pointing your head down to curve your spine inwards

5. slowly stand back up, bringing your feet back in towards the wall

6. repeat this 5-8 times

The aim is to feel this stretch along the center of your back and at the back of your ribs, though you may feel it to the sides too. Avoid pushing your hips away from the wall, instead of stepping backward, as this will transfer the bend to your hips instead of your back.

If you find this too difficult to do, it can be adapted by using a chair. Sit in your chair with your feet at hip-width apart and forward, aiming to touch the floor.

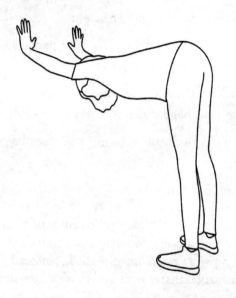

Puppy Stretch

Muscles targeted: rectus abdominis, oblique group, and to a lesser extent the pectoral group.

Step by step:

1. stand facing the wall with your feet hip-width apart

2. raise both arms above your head and bend them at the elbows to place your palms on the back of your head

3. touch your elbows to the wall

4. step backward away from the wall and lean forwards, keeping your head up to curve your spine outwards

5. hold for 30-60 seconds

Your hips will naturally move away from the wall as you do this. If you feel comfortable deepening the stretch, you can also allow your hips to tilt forward, or increase the distance between yourself and the wall.

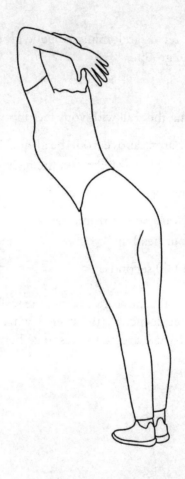

Chapter 7:

Lower Body Wall Stretches

Calf Stretch

Muscles targeted: gastrocnemius, soleus, flexor digitorum and digitorum brevis, abductor digiti minimi, abductor hallucis, flexor hallucis longus and hallucis brevis, and plantaris.

Step by step:

1. stand facing the wall at arm's length away, with your feet hip-width apart

2. place both of your palms against the wall to support yourself

3. bring your left leg forward, pointing your toes to the ceiling

4. push the ball of your foot to the wall with your heel on the floor

5. keep your knee straight and lean forward, increasing bend at your ankle

6. hold this position for 30-60 seconds

7. carefully push away from the wall and stand back upright, before bringing your foot back to rest at hip-width as before

8. repeat for the opposite leg.

Try to keep the leg that isn't being stretched with your heel on the floor; this will help to keep you balanced and prevent you from toppling over. If you find this stretch too difficult for your balance, you can substitute it with the sitting calf stretch chair exercise in chapter 5.

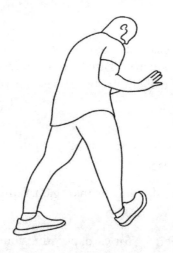

Calf/Achilles Stretch

Muscles targeted: soleus, plantaris, gastrocnemius, popliteus, tibialis posterior, flexor digitorum longus, and flexor hallucis longus.

Step by step:

1. face the wall, standing a little less than arm's length away, with your feet hip-width apart

2. place both hands on the wall to support you

3. step your left leg back as far as is comfortable for you

4. bend your right knee and lead your chest towards the wall

5. straighten your right leg and bring your left foot back to meet your right foot in the center.

6. repeat this with the opposite leg

7. alternate 5-8 times on each side

To get the best from this stretch, keep your back knee straight and your heel on the floor. If you are having problems keeping your heel to the floor, or it becomes painful, you can add a slight bend to your back knee, to reduce the difficulty of this stretch.

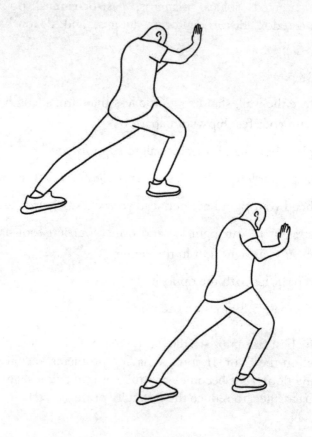

Standing Quad Stretch

Muscles targeted: quadriceps group, middle and upper sartorius, psoas major, iliacus, and tensor fasciae latae.

Step by step:

1. stand facing the wall, approximately a foot away, with your feet hip-distance apart

2. rest your right hand on the wall to support yourself

3. bend your left leg at the knee, bringing your ankle behind you

4. use your left hand to support your leg at the ankle

5. gently pull your ankle towards your bottom, increasing the bend of your knee

6. hold this position for 30-60 seconds

7. release your left leg, and return your foot to the floor

8. repeat with the opposite leg and arm

When you do this stretch, take care not to pull your leg out to the side, or to push your hips backward away from the wall. Both of these actions will transfer the stretch to your torso and hips, instead of stretching the front of your thighs as intended.

This stretch requires a good sense of balance; if you are unable to balance on one leg, even with the wall for support, you can adapt this stretch to be performed on the floor—Lay on your right side to stretch your left leg, and vice versa.

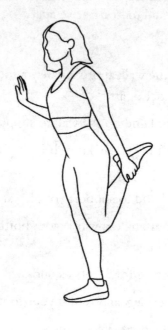

Standing Hamstring Stretch

Muscles targeted: hamstrings, gluteus maximus, gastrocnemius, and soleus.

Step by step:

1. stand facing away from the wall with your feet a couple of inches away from the wall

2. keep your feet flat on the floor and lean back until your bottom rests against the wall

3. breathe out and bend forwards, as if trying to touch the ground in front of you

4. rest your hands on your calves for support

5. hold this position for 30-60 seconds

When you have finished this stretch and return to standing upright, be sure to raise up slowly to prevent the onset of dizziness.

For best results, aim to keep your feet flat on the floor and your knees straight. However, if this is too difficult, you can reduce how low you reach toward the floor. Rest your hands above your knees instead of aiming for your calves. Never rest your weight directly on your knees, as this can cause overextension and injury.

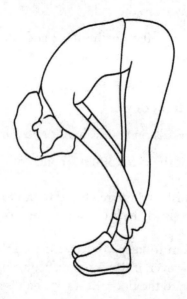

Figure Four

Muscles targeted: Gluteus group, piriformis, gemellus group, and obturator group.

Step by step:

1. lay on your back on the floor with your knees bent and toes touching the bottom of the wall

2. lift your right leg until you can place your foot flat against the wall

3. lift your left leg and cross your ankle over the top of your right knee

4. using your hands, gently push your left knee towards the wall

5. hold this position for 30-60 seconds

6. lower your feet back to the floor

7. repeat with the opposite leg - using the left leg to rest the right ankle

To get the best from this stretch, you want to aim to have the knee of your supporting leg at a 90-degree angle and the sole of the foot flat against the wall. You may need to shuffle closer to the wall to achieve this. Be sure not to cross the leg that you are stretching further than ankle to knee. You should also try to avoid bending your torso from side to side when you push your leg towards the wall, as this will reduce the effectiveness of the stretch.

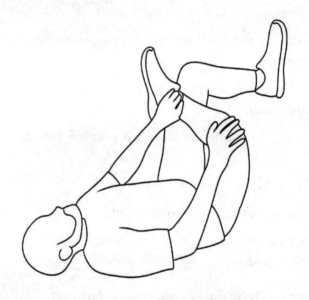

Happy Baby

Muscles targeted: gracilis, adductor group, pectineus, and middle artorius.

Step by step:

1. lay on your back, the floor with your knees bent and toes touching the bottom of the wall

2. lift both legs and place your feet flat against the wall

3. spread your feet until they are roughly shoulder-width apart

4. place your hands on your knees

5. gently pull your knees outwards, and down towards the floor as far as comfortable

6. hold this position for 30-60 seconds

Aim to rest the soles of your feet flat against the wall, with your knees bent at 90 degrees, you may need to shuffle towards the wall after you have lifted your legs to achieve this. You may also find that your toes will point slightly outwards while you do this, this is not a problem, but avoid allowing your ankles to roll over your foot so that your soles point towards each other.

If you find this too difficult, you can adapt by stretching one leg at a time. Leave your other leg resting with your foot flat on the floor and your knees bent.

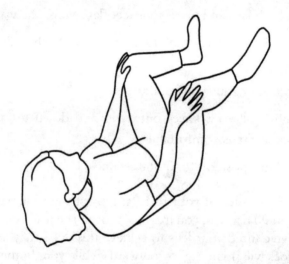

Chapter 8:

Upper Body Floor Stretches

Child's Pose

Muscles targeted: erector spinae group, latissimus dorsi, posterior deltoid, quadratus lumborum, multifidus, gluteus group, quadriceps group, tibialis anterior, extensor digitorum longus, extensor hallucis longus, intercostals, and splenius group.

Step by step:

1. kneel on the floor with your knees hip-width apart

2. lean forward and place both palms flat on the floor in front of you

3. keep your palms touching the floor and sit back towards your ankles

4. breathe out and reach your arms forwards to deepen the stretch of your spine

5. hold this position for 30-60 seconds

If possible, aim to touch your forehead to the floor. You can deepen the effect of this stretch by pushing your bottom further towards your ankles. This stretch is popular in yoga and is a great tool for relaxation. The pose is close to the fetal position, allows for deep breathing, and is considered the best position to rest in.

If you are finding this position difficult, you can adapt it by opening your knees to create a space for your torso to drop into.

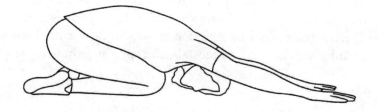

Tricep Stretch

Muscles targeted: triceps brachii, posterior deltoid, teres minor and major, and latissimus dorsi.

Step by step:

1. sit comfortably on the floor with your legs out in front of you

2. raise your left arm above your head, then bend it at the elbow to touch the space on your back between your shoulder blades

3. raise your right arm up and over your head, placing your hand on your left elbow

4. gently pull your left elbow back past your left ear

5. hold this position for 30-60 seconds

6. repeat with your opposite arm

When you pull your elbow backward, also aim down towards the floor behind you in a curve. Imagine it like a compass where your elbow is the pencil drawing the curve, and your shoulder is the center point.

If you are finding this stretch difficult, you can reduce the intensity by placing your hand in-line with the back of your neck, instead of reaching down between your shoulder blades. Since this stretch is intended for your arm and upper torso, you may also wish to sit cross-legged to feel more comfortable if you are struggling.

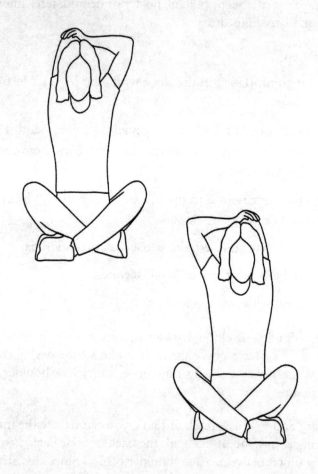

Cat-Cow Stretch

This stretch is a dynamic stretch where you will be moving between two different poses. Always remember that your movements should be at a slow and steady pace, if you rush them you won't experience the potential benefits.

Muscles targeted in cat pose: quadratus lumborum, erector spinae, trapezius, rhomboid, latissimus dorsi, splenius group, to a lesser extent, the flexor diditorum superficialis, and palmaris longus.

Muscles targeted in cow pose: gluteus group, rectus abdominis, oblique group, sternocleidomastoid, longissimus capitis, scalene group, and to a lesser extent, the flexor diditorum superficialis, palmaris longus, pectoral group, and serratus anterior.

Step by step:

1. kneel on the floor with your knees hip-width apart

2. lean forward to place both palms on the floor with your fingers pointing towards the wall in front of you, shoulder-width apart

3. breathe out while contracting your stomach muscles to curve your spine up towards the ceiling - this is cat pose

4. drop your head down to continue the curve of your spine right through your neck

5. breathe in, while releasing your stomach muscles, allowing your abdomen area to drop towards the floor. This is the cow pose

6. lift your head and be sure that your face is pointing forwards

7. repeat, alternating between the cat and cow poses 5-8 times each way

Imagine your spine as a 'c' shape and alternate the direction that the 'c' curves with each movement. If you achieve a deep curve, you will notice that your shoulders will round as you enter the cat pose and open as you enter the cow pose. As you become more practiced at this stretching technique, you will learn to move your back, head, and shoulders simultaneously. Avoid allowing your elbows to rotate outward, as this puts unnecessary pressure on the joint and can be damaging. You will be putting approximately half the weight of your torso through your arms during this stretch.

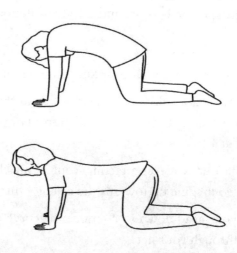

Lying T Twist

Muscles targeted: oblique group, transverse abdominis, quadratus lumborum, erector spinae group, latissimus dorsi, and to a lesser extent, the pectoralis group, serratus anterior, and intercostals.

Step by step:

1. lay on your back, resting your arms out to the sides at shoulder level

2. lift both of your legs together, creating a 90-degree angle at both your hips and knees

3. keep your upper torso in place, breathe out and twist the lower torso to the left, until you can touch the floor with the outer thigh of your left leg

4. breathe in while you twist back to center, raising your leg.

5. breathe out and twist your lower torso to the right until you can feel your right outer thigh touch the floor

6. breathe in again and lift your legs, returning your torso to center

7. repeat, alternating from side to side 5-8 times each way

Though a slight lift is normal, aim to keep your shoulders touching the floor throughout the movement. You should be rocking your hips from side to side against the floor to achieve a smooth twist. Remember to move slowly and steadily; dropping your legs too quickly can cause pain in your lower back.

If you are finding it too difficult to touch the floor each time you twist to the side, you can adapt it by keeping your feet flat on the floor with your knees bent. As you turn to the side, your feet will naturally lift; this is fine but keep contact with the floor to support yourself as you twist. This way, if you can't make the full twist, your legs will have support and won't put extra pressure on your stomach muscles to keep your feet in the air.

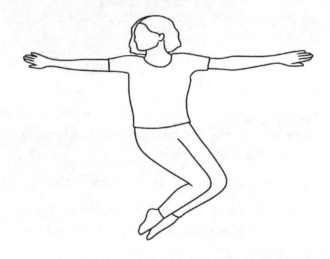

Abdominal Stretch

Muscles targeted: rectus abdominis, and the obliques group.

Step by step:

1. lay face down on the floor

2. place both palms on the floor next to your shoulders

3. keep your hips on the floor while you straighten your arms, lifting your chest up off the floor

4. bend your arms at the elbow to gently lower yourself back to the floor

5. repeat 5-8 times

Avoid allowing your elbow to rotate outwards, and keep your head up and facing forwards whenever you lift yourself up. Keep your hips and thighs in contact with the floor as much as possible. If you are finding this stretch too difficult, you can adapt by reducing how far you lift your chest and keeping a slight bend in your elbows.

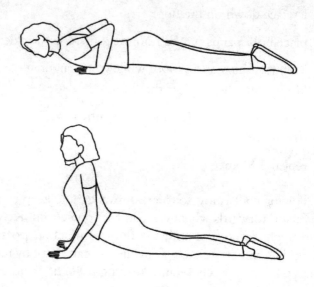

Chapter 9:

Lower Body Floor Stretches

90 - 90 Stretch

Muscles targeted: tensor fascia latae, rectus femoris, vastus group, pectineus, sartorius, anterior, iliacus, adductor group, piriformis, gemellus group, obturator internus, quadratus femoris, gluteus group, latissimus dorsi, and erector spinae group.

Step by step:

1. sit on the floor with your legs crossed in front of you

2. allow your left leg to form a 90-degree angle at the knee, with your outer knee and ankle touching the floor

3. uncross your right leg

4. rotate your right leg so that your inner ankle is towards the floor.

5. bring your right foot behind you, creating another 90-degree angle at your knee

6. grasp your left foot with your right hand

7. breathe out, and lean forwards. Gently push your torso towards the floor in front of you

8. hold this position for 30-60 seconds

9. sit up and bring your right foot back around in front of you

10. repeat with your legs in the opposite position

This is a complex stretch as it rotates your hips in opposite directions, one internal and one external, at the same time. The key to getting the correct positioning of your legs is to ensure that the thigh of the back leg is in line with your arm on the same side of your body when you lift it out to your side. For the front leg, ensure your thigh is pointing straight out in front of you.

If you find this stretch too difficult it can be adapted by either reducing, or removing the forward lean. Instead, concentrate on keeping an upright posture, with your torso facing forwards. Getting your legs into the correct position alone can be a tough task if you are not used to performing inward rotation of your hips.

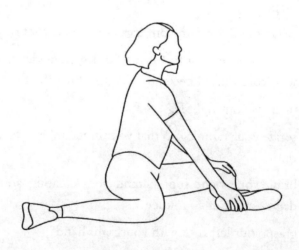

Frog Stretch

Muscles targeted: gracilis, hip adductor group, mid-sartorius, and to a lesser extent, the gluteus group.

Step by step:

1. kneel on the floor with your knees hip-width apart

2. lean forwards and place your palms on the floor in front of you, with your hands shoulder-width apart

3. one at a time, bend your elbow to 90 degrees and drop down, laying your forearm across the floor in front of you

4. one at a time, move your knees outwards, dropping your hips towards the floor

5. hold this position for 30-60 seconds

Try to keep your toes pointing down to the floor while you do this stretch. If you feel like you are able to increase the intensity of the stretch, you can move your knees further apart. The further you lower yourself to the ground, the more difficult it will become.

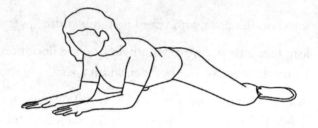

Lunging Hip Flexor Stretch

Muscles targeted: vastus group, sartorius group, rectus femoris, psoas major, iliacus, tensor fasciae latae, anterior gluteus medius, and pectineus.

Step by step:

1. kneel on the floor with your knees hip-width apart and your toes pointing down to the floor

2. raise your left leg, placing your foot flat on the floor in front of you, bending the knee at a 90-degree angle

3. rest your hands at the top of your thighs, and push your hips forwards in a lunging motion

4. hold this position for 30-60 seconds

5. repeat with your legs in the opposite positions

Be sure to keep a straight back and tall posture as you push forwards, if you curl your torso forward you will lose the effect of the stretch. It is also important to keep the knee of your back leg touching the floor as far as possible to ensure that you have a stable base to stretch from.

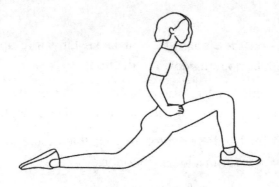

Knee To Chest Stretch

Muscles targeted: erector spinae group, multifidus, latissimus dorsi, semitendinosus, semimembranosus, and gluteus group.

Step by step:

1. lay flat on your back, on the floor
2. lift both your legs, bending at the knees
3. grasp each leg just below the knee

4. gently pull your knees into your chest

5. hold this position for 30-60 seconds

The aim of this stretch is to achieve a curve of the spine all the way through the lower back, the further into your chest that you pull your knees, the deeper the stretch will be. Avoid allowing your torso to twist, and keep your head flat on the floor as far as possible.

If you find it too difficult, you can adapt this stretch by raising one leg at a time, but be sure to do both sides.

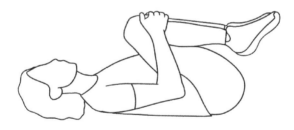

Seated Hamstring Stretch

Muscles targeted: gastrocnemius, plantaris, soleus, semitendinosus, and semimembranosus.

Step by step:

1. sit on the floor with your legs straight out in front of you

2. move your feet apart as far as is comfortable to create a 'v' shape with your legs

3. breathe out and lean over your left leg

4. grasp your left leg just above the ankle and gently push your torso further downwards

5. hold this position for 30-60 seconds

6. sit upright and center yourself

7. breathe out and lean over your right leg

8. grasp your right leg just above the ankle and gently push your torso further downwards

9. hold this position for 30-60 seconds

If you spend a lot of time standing you may find this stretch uncomfortable, if it begins to hurt at all then pull back. If you find it too difficult to complete, you can reduce the intensity of the stretch by bending at the knee on the leg you aren't currently stretching, tucking your foot towards your hips.

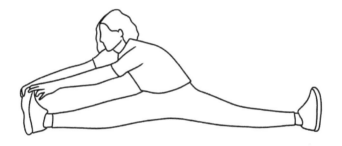

Chapter 10:

Frozen Shoulder-Easing Aches and Pains Associated With Shoulder Stiffness

Healthy Shoulder Structure and Movement

The shoulder joint is the point at the top of your arm where the scapula, clavicle, and humerus bones meet the shoulder blade, collar bone, and upper arm bone. Although not considered to be a part of the shoulder joint itself, the joint between the clavicle and sternum can also affect the proper function of the shoulder.

The acromioclavicular joint is the point in the shoulder where the clavicle meets the scapula at a bony outcrop called the acromion. You can find this area with your fingers by sliding them across your clavicle, outwards from the center of your chest, until you feel the protrusion where the two bones meet at the top of your shoulder. If you keep your fingers there and make circles with your shoulder, you will be able to feel this joint opening and closing.

Ligaments often have long names and can be difficult to remember, but it isn't necessary to worry about memorizing them all; I have only included the names so that you can have a point of reference if your health care provider has told you that these are the ones affected by your condition. The acromioclavicular area of your shoulder is stabilized by the following ligaments: the extracapsular accessory ligament, and the coracoclavicular ligament. Strength is also lent to this joint by the trapezius and deltoid muscles as they cross over it. However, this joint doesn't have any muscles of its own, directly contributing to its movement; it moves as a consequence of active movement in the glenohumeral joint - also known as the true shoulder joint.

The glenohumeral joint is the area in the shoulder where the humerus and scapula meet, and is classified as a ball and socket joint. Unlike the acromioclavicular joint, the glenohumeral joint can not be felt from the outside, this is due to it being surrounded by many muscles.

The glenohumeral joint is made between the glenoid fossa-a curved indent in the scapula - and the head of the humerus-the rounded topmost surface of the humerus. It is stabilized by two groups of ligaments, the capsular ligaments, and the accessory ligaments. The capsular group includes the following ligaments:

- superior glenohumeral ligament: connecting the top of the glenoid fossa and the top of the lesser tubercle - a bony outcrop on the front of the humerus

- middle glenohumeral ligament: connecting just below the superior ligament on the glenoid fossa, and front of the lesser tubercle

- inferior glenohumeral ligament: connecting the lower front edge of the glenoid fossa, and the underneath of the neck of the humerus

The accessory ligaments include the following:

- coracohumeral ligament: joining the coracoid process - a bony outcrop at the back of the scapula - from where it splits to join two areas of the humerus, at the lesser tubercle, and greater tubercle - at the back of the humerus

- coracoacromial ligament: spanning between the two outcrops of the scapula - the acromion and coracoid process

Due to its complexity, the shoulder is capable of movement in several directions. Healthy movement of your upper limbs at the shoulder is driven by a combination of movement around the shoulder joint, and the ability to independently move the scapula over the back of the rib cage. Movements available to the shoulder include:

- shoulder flexion: raising your arm out in front of you

- shoulder extension: pushing your arm back behind you

- shoulder abduction: raising your arm out to the side, away from your body

- shoulder adduction: lowering your arm back towards your torso

- internal or medial rotation: twisting your upper arm in towards your body

- external or lateral rotation: twisting your upper arm outwards towards the back of your body

The shoulder is also able to perform the following movements of the scapula:

- retraction: the scapula stays upright and is pulled in towards the spine

- protraction: the scapula stays upright and is pulled forwards around the curve of the rib cage

- elevation: the scapula moves directly upwards

- depression: the scapula is pulled downwards

- lateral rotation: the scapula twists, creating an angle where the top outer edge raises and the bottom moves outwards around the rib cage

- medial rotation: the action where the scapula is returned to its resting point after lateral rotation

These movements are all initiated and controlled by a complex network of muscles surrounding the upper arm, chest, and shoulder. As with ligaments, your doctor or physical therapist may tell you that you have certain muscles that are affected by your condition. For this reason, I have included the names of muscles targeted during each stretch listed in this book, so that you can be confident that you are choosing the right set of stretches, to target the tightened areas that you personally want to improve.

However, if you are told that you would benefit from strengthening certain muscles, you will typically need to be working in the opposite movements to those in which they are stretched. Below is a quick reference table of the muscles surrounding your shoulder and the movement directions that will cause them to perform the work of the movement, therefore helping you to strengthen them.

Muscle Name	Working Movement Direction
Rhomboid major	Retraction/Medial rotation of scapula
Rhomboid minor	Retraction/Medial rotation of scapula

Muscle Name	Working Movement Direction
Trapezius	Retraction/Elevation/Depression/Lateral rotation of scapula
Serratus anterior	Protraction/Lateral rotation of scapula
Pectoralis minor	Protraction/Depression/Medial rotation of scapula
Pectoralis major	Flexion/Extension/Adduction/Internal rotation of the arm
Levator scapulae	Elevation/Medial rotation of scapula
Supraspinatus	Abduction
Deltoid	Abduction/Flexion/Extension/Internal rotation of the arm/External rotation of the arm
Biceps brachii	Flexion
Coracobrachialis	Flexion/Adduction
Latissimus dorsi	Extension/Adduction/Internal rotation of the arm
Teres major	Extension/Adduction/Internal rotation of the arm

Muscle Name	Working Movement Direction
Teres minor	External rotation of the arm
Triceps	Extension
Subscapularis	Internal rotation of the arm
Infraspinatus	External rotation of the arm

What Is a Frozen Shoulder?

Frozen shoulder is a painful condition affecting the shoulder joint and surrounding area that results in reduced ROM. The level of pain varies from person to person, and may be dependent on the level of progression of the condition too.

Typically the condition will involve three stages, each potentially lasting a number of months:

1. Freezing: the shoulder will become stiffer as time progresses and pain increases when attempting to move the joint. Sufferers often report an increase in this pain at night, and an inability to sleep on the affected side. This stage can last for 2-9 months.

2. Frozen: this stage is marked by a reduction in pain, but severe limitation in ROM. Sufferers find it increasingly difficult to move the joint and often report an inability to raise the arm above their head, or place it behind their backs. This stage can last for 4-12 months.

3. Thawing or resolution: this stage can last from 12-42 months. During this time, the shoulder will gradually regain its mobility. There is sometimes a recurrence of pain in this stage, but it is notably less severe than in stage one.

The exact cause of a frozen shoulder is not certain. However, it is agreed that the joint capsule stiffens, and scarring occurs in the soft tissues supporting the joint. It is more likely to affect people who have undergone surgeries that cause immobilization for an extended time during recovery, and those with diabetes, thyroid conditions, or cardiovascular disease.

Typically the condition affects people older than 40 and is more likely to affect women than men (Mayo Foundation for Medical Education and Research, 2020). Treatment for the condition is another thing that varies from person to person, but is typically aimed at joint mobilization and other physical therapies. Occasionally sufferers will receive corticosteroid injections, and in a small number of cases will require orthopedic surgery to release the joint capsule.

Cautions

The exercises in this chapter are intended to relieve aches and pains; they should never create more pain while you are performing them. Remember that stretching should be enjoyable and relax both your body, and mind.

These stretches are a tool to help alleviate your pain; they are not a cure or a diagnosis. It is important that you contact your primary care doctor, or other health care professional if you have any concerns about the health of your body. If you have already received a diagnosis for any of the conditions below, be sure to regularly review with your doctor, and consult them before starting a new exercise program.

Stretches to Manage a Frozen Shoulder

The following stretches are designed to reduce pain and improve ROM in the shoulder; they can also be used as a preventative for people who may be at risk of developing a frozen shoulder.

You will need an exercise bar to aid these stretches; if you do not own one, a mop or broom handle can also be used. Don't push your shoulder so far that it increases your pain; pull back if this happens. Be patient with yourself; it can take time to repair a frozen shoulder.

Shoulder Flexion

Muscles targeted: posterior deltoid, teres group, rhomboid, trapezius group, latissimus dorsi, and triceps brachii.

Step by step:

1. stand with your feet hip-width apart

2. grasp your exercise bar over the end with your hand on the affected side

3. grasp the bar with your other hand so that your hands are roughly shoulder-width apart

4. turn the bar to a vertical position, so that your healthy arm is on the bottom

5. use your healthy arm to gently push the bar upwards, doing the work of raising your affected arm towards the ceiling, as far as is comfortable for you

6. lower the bar to rest your arms

7. repeat 5-8 times

If you have a severe restriction of your ROM or are experiencing the freezing stage, you may not be able to move your affected shoulder very far. This is normal, and your aim is to increase your ROM over time with this stretch. Avoid pushing your affected arm outwards and to the side. You should be aiming for a straight up and down movement of the arm.

If you have difficulty standing for extended periods of time, this stretch can also be performed while sitting. Be sure to allow for free clearance of the bar that you use in front of the seat.

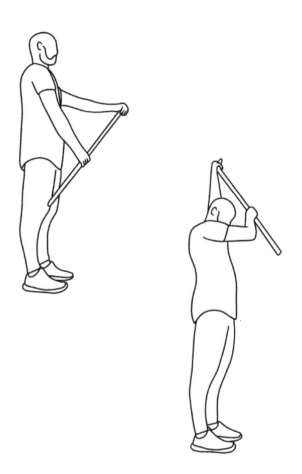

Shoulder Extension

Muscles targeted: anterior deltoid, pectoralis group, subclavius, biceps brachii, and Coracobrachialis.

Step by step:

1. stand with your feet hip-width apart

2. grasp your exercise bar over the end with your hand on your healthy side

3. grasp the bar with your other hand so that your hands are shoulder-width apart

4. hold the bar horizontally to the side of your torso, on the side of your affected arm, so that your healthy arm is out in front of you

5. use your healthy arm to gently push the bar behind you, doing the work of raising your affected arm towards the ceiling behind your back, as far as is comfortable for you

6. pull the bar back to your front to rest your arms

7. repeat 5-8 times

The action you are looking for is similar to rowing a boat with a single-sided paddle so that your affected arm moves gently behind your torso and upwards at the same time. Be aware that the normal ROM for most people in this direction is below shoulder height, so don't try to force it straight up like you would be able to do if you were circling it forwards. However, with a frozen shoulder, this can be significantly reduced; any amount of backward motion behind the torso is good as long as it remains pain-free. If you do have a limited ROM, it can be tempting to allow your torso to twist or your hips to bend forwards, avoid doing this, as it is transferring the movement to the wrong area of your body.

If you are finding it difficult to perform this stretch while standing, you can adapt it to be done while sitting in a chair.

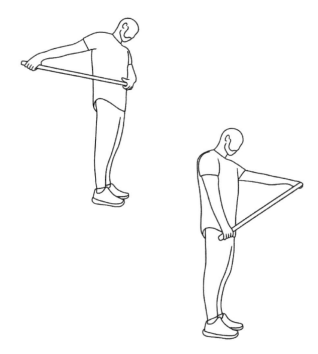

Shoulder Abduction

Muscles targeted: latissimus dorsi, teres group, deltoid group, pectoralis major, subscapularis, and triceps brachii.

Step by step:

1. stand with your feet hip-width apart
2. grasp your exercise bar with both hands, a little more than shoulder-width apart
3. hold the bar horizontally in front of you
4. bend the elbow of your healthy arm to gently push the bar up and out to the side, doing the work of raising your affected arm away from your torso
5. pull the bar back down to rest your arms
6. repeat 5-8 times

Aim to raise your affected arm out to the side as far as is comfortable for you. Maintaining steady breathing is particularly important during this stretch, as holding your breath will tense the muscles in your ribcage and increase the level of difficulty. To get the best results from this stretch, concentrate on the action of bending your healthy arm at the elbow. If you start to push the exercise bar without introducing this bend, you will twist the torso and lessen its effectiveness.

This stretch is not suitable to be performed in a chair.

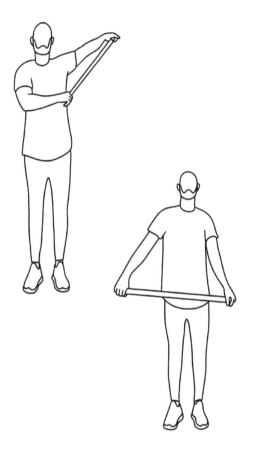

External Rotation

Muscles targeted: deltoid anterior, latissimus dorsi, pectoralis major, teres major, and subscapularis.

Step by step:

1. stand with your feet hip-width apart

2. grasp your exercise bar over the end with your hand on the affected side

3. grasp the bar with your other hand so that your hands are roughly shoulder-width apart

4. hold the bar horizontally in front of you

5. on your affected side, bend your arm to 90-degree at the elbow, and tuck your elbow into the side of your torso

6. use your healthy arm to gently push the bar sideways towards your affected side, doing the work of turning your affected arm outwards away from the body, as far as is comfortable for you

7. return the bar to the center to rest your arms

8. repeat 5-8 times

The elbow tuck is key to performing this stretch effectively. You should avoid any sort of lifting motion in your affected shoulder, aiming instead for a twist of the upper arm away from the torso.

If you have difficulty standing to perform this stretch, it can be adapted to be done while sitting in a chair.

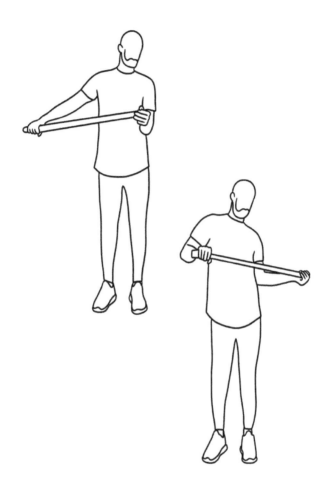

Internal Rotation

Muscles targeted: deltoid posterior, infraspinatus, teres minor, and coracobrachialis.

Step by step:

1. stand with your feet hip-width apart

2. grasp your exercise bar over the end with your hand on the affected side

3. grasp the bar with your other hand so that your hands are roughly shoulder-width apart

4. hold the bar horizontally in front of you

5. on your affected side, bend your arm to 90 degrees at the elbow, and tuck your elbow into the side of your torso

6. use your healthy arm to gently pull the bar sideways towards your healthy side, doing the work of turning your affected arm inwards towards the body, as far as is comfortable for you

7. return the bar to the center to rest your arms

8. repeat 5-8 times

As with external rotation, the key for internal rotation is the elbow tuck. Aim for a twisting motion in the upper arm of your affected side. If you find it difficult to remain standing while performing this stretch, it can be adapted to be done while sitting in a chair.

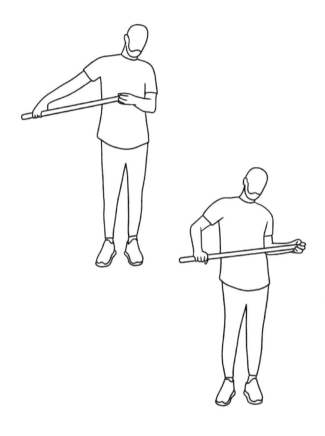

Chapter 11:

Sciatica-Easing Aches and Pains Associated With the Impinged Nerve

Healthy Lumbar Spine and Hip Structure, Movement, and the Sciatic Nerve

The spine at the lower back is made up of five lumbar vertebrae, and terminates with the sacrum. The joints between each vertebra are known as the intervertebral joints and although each bone does make contact with the one below, the largest surfaces of the bones are separated by a fibrous cousin called an intervertebral disc, which is anchored to the bones above and below it; these discs have a richly hydrated center and are thickest in the lumbar region.

Intervertebral discs are wedge-shaped, which allows them to create the natural curves of the spine; in the lumbar region, the widest section is towards the front of the spine, creating the deep forwards curve of the lower back. The discs act as both cushions for the upper body weight, and dictate the direction of movement for each joint in the lower back. When you hear the phrase 'slipped disc', it is excessive movement or damage to the intervertebral discs, causing them to bulge out or rupture, that is being referred to.

Since the lumbar region of the spine needs to be able to support the weight of the whole upper body, the ligaments in the area are very densely packed with fibrous tissue. The front of the spine is supported by the anterior longitudinal ligament, which runs the entire length of the spine. In the lower back, it anchors onto the sacrum, and can be up to an inch wide. This ligament is responsible for preventing each lumbar vertebrae from sliding forwards and off the surface of the one below. At the back of the spine the area is supported by the posterior longitudinal ligament. This ligament is generally not as strong as its anterior counterpart; it can be around two-thirds the thickness and as small as a third of an inch in width too.

Though the pair of longitudinal ligaments do the majority of the work in stabilizing the spine, there are also some accessory ligaments found connecting the bony protrusions at the back of each vertebra. The supraspinous ligament runs the length of the spine connecting the outermost surfaces of these protrusions, and the interspinous ligaments are found in between each vertebrae spanning the gap between each protrusion. There is also a third type of accessory ligament between each vertebra that is usually considered insignificant, but becomes stronger in the lumbar region. These ligaments are called the intertransverse ligaments, and span the gaps between smaller bony protrusions on either side of the central one at the back of the vertebrae. Intertransverse ligaments prevent the vertebrae from moving too far in either sideways direction, which is why you get less lateral movement in the lower back than in other areas of the spine.

Despite the heavy lifting required by the spine, it is still capable of a tremendous amount of movement. It can move large areas by dividing the total movement into small petitions at each intervertebral joint. As a result, the spine is able to perform the following types of movement:

- flexion: the action of bending forwards

- extension: the action of bending backwards

- lateral flexion: the action of bending to either side

- rotation: the action of twisting the torso

I mentioned that the lumbar region of the spine terminates at the bottom with the sacrum. This is important as the curve of the sacrum contributes to the creation of the pelvic girdle, this is a region where the lower body organs are held, such as the bladder and reproductive organs. The sacrum joins with each pelvis bone on either side, at an area known as the sacroiliac joint, though this is not a part of the hip joint, it still has an important role to play in the healthy function of the legs since it is responsible for transferring the weight from the spine around to the lower limbs. Ligaments supporting the spines connection to the sacrum, and pelvis, additional to the longitudinal ligaments include the following:

- iliolumbar ligament: connects the top of the pelvis to the lumbar vertebrae

- lateral lumbosacral ligament: starting next to the vertebral connection of the iliolumbar ligament, connecting the spine to the top edge of the sacrum

The true hip joint is the area at the top of the leg where the pelvis and femur meet. Similar to the shoulder, the hip joint is classified as a ball joint. However, due to the large difference in weight that the joint must be capable of supporting, the adjoining surfaces of the bone are much larger. The ball, or head, of the femur, meets the pelvis at a deep spherical notch that forms the socket of the joint, known as the acetabulum. The hip joint is not able to be felt from the outside, though if you slide your hands from the hollow of your buttocks around the side of your thigh, you will feel a bony protrusion called the greater trochanter. This protrusion is the top, outwardly facing, edge of the femur, which is adjacent but a little lower than the hip joint itself.

As I'm sure you will have noticed, the amount of weight that a joint needs to bear is a direct correlation factor to the strength that the ligaments of the area must provide. The hip is no exception to this rule, with several ligaments joining the pelvis to the spine, and the femur to the pelvis. Ligaments in this area fall into two categories, capsular ligaments, which surround the outside of the joint capsule, and intracapsular ligaments, which are inside the joint capsule itself.

The capsular ligaments do the heavy work for stabilizing the hip and include the following:

- iliofemoral ligament: connecting the ilium of the pelvis to the front of the femur at the trochanter. This ligament is very wide and considered the strongest in the hip joint

- pubofemoral ligament: connecting the lower frontal area of the pelvis to the femur below the iliofemoral ligament

- ischiofemoral ligament: connecting the back area of the acetabulum to the neck of the femur

The intracapsular ligaments are smaller and include the following:

- transverse ligament of the acetabulum: connects the lower open edges of the acetabulum to form a complete socket into which the femur connects, whilst allowing blood vessels and nerves to pass though the joint

- ligamentum teres: connects the head of the femur to the upper edge of the transverse ligament

Despite being developed to be much more structurally firm than the shoulder joint, the hip is still capable of a large ROM. Movement directions available to the hip include the following:

- flexion: bending forwards, or bringing the knee up to the chest

- extension: putting the leg out behind the torso

- abduction: lifting the leg out to the side of the torso

- adduction: returning the leg to the center line, or crossing one leg in front of the other

- medial or internal rotation: the inward twisting of the knee in relation to the pelvis

- lateral or external rotation: the outward twisting of the knee in relation to the pelvis

If your doctor or physical therapist tells you that you have particular muscles that are tight, you can refer to the targeted muscles listed with each stretch in this book. However, if they tell you that you could benefit from strengthening a particular muscle, this will often need a movement that is opposite to the one that would stretch that muscle. I have provided the quick reference table below to show you which muscles are responsible for doing the active work of each movement type and therefore, which movement direction will help to strengthen them.

Muscle Name	Working Movement Direction
Rectus abdominis	Torso flexion/Torso lateral flexion
External oblique	Torso flexion/Torso rotation/Torso lateral flexion

Muscle Name	Working Movement Direction
Internal oblique	Torso flexion/Torso rotation/Torso lateral flexion
Psoas minor	Torso flexion
Psoas major	Torso flexion/Hip flexion/Hip medial rotation
Quadratus lumborum	Torso extension/Torso lateral flexion
Multifidus	Torso extension/Torso rotation/Torso lateral flexion
Semispinalis	Torso extension/Torso rotation
Erector spinae	Torso extension/Torso lateral flexion
Rotatores	Torso rotation
Intertransversarii	Torso lateral flexion
Gluteus maximus	Hip extension/Hip abduction/Hip lateral rotation
Gluteus medius	Hip abduction/Hip medial rotation
Gluteus minimus	Hip abduction/Hip medial rotation
Hamstrings (Semitendinosus/Semi	Hip extension

Muscle Name	Working Movement Direction
membranosus/Biceps femoris)	
Tensor fascia lata	Hip abduction/Hip medial rotation
Adductor magnus	Hip adduction
Adductor longus	Hip adduction
Adductor brevis	Hip adduction
Gracilis	Hip adduction
Pectineus	Hip adduction/Hip flexion
Iliacus	Hip flexion/Hip medial rotation
Rectus femoris	Hip flexion
Sartorius	Hip flexion
Piriformis	Hip lateral rotation
Obturator internus	Hip lateral rotation
Gemellus superior	Hip lateral rotation
Gemellus inferior	Hip lateral rotation
Quadratus femoris	Hip lateral rotation

Muscle Name	Working Movement Direction
Obturator externus	Hip lateral rotation

Now you know what contributes to healthily functioning mechanics of the lower back and hip joints, I'd like to explain a little on the pathway of the sciatic nerve before moving on to discuss the condition of sciatica itself. The sciatic nerve is the largest nerve in the body; it branches out from your spine in the lumbar region and tracks down the whole leg before entering the foot. It's a long and complex nerve, but its path is important in understanding the areas that can be affected and show symptoms of sciatica.

The sciatic nerve actually consists of two major nerves that travel along the leg together in the same nerve sheath, the common fibular nerve and the tibial nerve. The common fibular nerve has roots originating from the spinal cord that emerge out between the vertebrae between the fourth and fifth lumbar vertebrae and the first and second sacral divisions. Similarly, the tibial nerve leaves the spinal cord in multiple places, also starting with the fourth lumbar vertebrae but continuing to the third sacral division. These nerves together, forming the sciatic nerve, leave the pelvis below the piriformis muscle. It runs between the quadriceps and the adductor muscles, then down the back of the thigh, around two-thirds of the way down, the two contributing nerves split out into their separate parts.

The common fibular nerve usually terminates on the outer side of the calf a couple of inches below the knee. In contrast, the tibial nerve goes on to run the whole length of the leg at the back of the calf. Near the ankle, it moves over to the inner side of the foot, from where it branches further into the plantar nerves of the foot.

What Is Sciatica?

Sciatica is a painful condition associated with back and leg pain. Impingement or compression of this nerve results in sciatic pain along any part of the nerve or its constituent parts.

Symptoms can vary from person to person, it is possible for both legs to be affected, but most often, it will only be present on one side. The key marker that highlights the difference between back pain, and sciatica, is accompanying pain in the leg. Often the pain is described by sufferers as starting in the back and radiating out to the buttocks and thigh. Though, it is possible to feel pain anywhere along the length of the sciatic nerve with this condition. The type of pain also varies, from a near-constant dull pain to a sudden intense pain, often described as a shock down the leg.

There are also a number of other symptoms associated with sciatica, including numbness, burning, tingling, and weakness in the leg. Not everyone affected will experience all of the symptoms, but on the flip side, some people will experience many; for some, this may even be different symptoms in different locations of the leg at once.

There can be many causes of sciatica, but they all result in compression of the sciatic nerve or its roots near the spine, which results in symptom onset. The most common causes are herniated discs or bone spurs in the lumbar spine, a narrowing of the opening in the spine where the sciatic nerve branches away from the spinal cord, or inflammation of the surrounding muscles.

Sciatica most commonly occurs later in life due to age-related conditions of the spine; however, traumatic injury can also trigger it. There are some other risk factors involved in developing the condition too. Those who are obese are at higher risk due to additional stress on the spine, but occupational hazards can also increase the risk of developing the condition. You are more likely to suffer from sciatica if you have worked in an occupation that requires you to twist your back or regularly carry heavy loads. Vehicle operatives and drivers are also at increased risk due to prolonged periods of sitting which can compress the nerve in the thigh as well as negatively affect the posture of the lower back.

There are a few red flags to look out for if you are experiencing symptoms of sciatica, if you experience symptoms for more than 3 months, then a trip to your primary care doctor is recommended. Immediate medical attention should be sought if you experience any of the following along with sciatic pain:

- loss of bowel or bladder function

- loss of feeling in the back or leg

- sudden onset of weakness in the leg

- the onset of pain is sudden, severe, or immediately following a traumatic injury - such as a road traffic collision.

Regular exercise can reduce the likelihood of developing sciatica, and stretches to improve the mobility of the spine are commonly prescribed soft therapies for the condition, which is expected to resolve in a few months for most sufferers. I recommend that you continue to use these stretches after the condition resolves to minimize the risks of a recurrence. In rare cases, if the pain becomes chronic, or is associated with injury then surgical intervention may be required.

The following stretches can be used as a preventative to reduce risk, or as a therapeutic exercise to alleviate pain. Remember that stretching should never cause pain or intensify existing pain, if you experience this, then you need to discontinue and seek medical advice.

Cautions

The exercises in this chapter are intended to relieve aches and pains; they should never create more pain while you are performing them. Remember that stretching should be enjoyable and relax both your body and mind.

These stretches are a tool to help alleviate your pain; they are not a cure or a diagnosis. It is important that you contact your primary care doctor, or other health care professional if you have any concerns about the health of your body. If you have already received a diagnosis for any of the conditions below, be sure to regularly review with your doctor, and consult them before starting a new exercise program.

Stretches to Manage Sciatica

Cat-Cow Pose

Here is a reminder of the targeted muscles and, step by step, of the cat-cow poses. Additional detail can be found in chapter eight: Upper Body Floor Stretches.

Muscles targeted in cat pose: quadratus lumborum, erector spinae, trapezius, rhomboid, latissimus dorsi, splenius group, to a lesser extent, the flexor diditorum superficialis, and palmaris longus.

Muscles targeted in cow pose: gluteus group, rectus abdominis, oblique group, sternocleidomastoid, longissimus capitis, scalene group, and to a lesser extent, the flexor diditorum superficialis, palmaris longus, pectoral group, and serratus anterior.

Step by step:

1. kneel on the floor with your knees hip-width apart

2. lean forward to place both palms on the floor with your fingers pointing towards the wall in front of you, shoulder-width apart

3. breathe out while contracting your stomach muscles to curve your spine up towards the ceiling - this is cat pose.

4. drop your head down to continue the curve of your spine all the way through your neck

5. breathe in, while releasing your stomach muscles, allowing your abdomen area to drop towards the floor. - this is the cow pose.

6. lift your head and be sure that your face is pointing forwards

7. repeat, alternating between the cat and cow poses 5-8 times each way

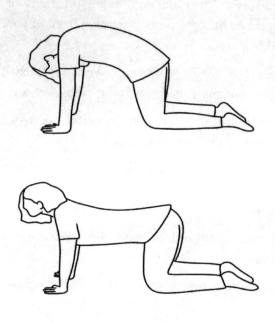

Abdominal Stretch

Here is a reminder of the targeted muscles and, step by step, of the abdominal stretch. Additional detail can be found in chapter eight: Upper Body Floor Stretches.

Muscles targeted: rectus abdominis, and the obliques group.

Step by step:

1. lay face down on the floor

2. place both palms on the floor next to your shoulders

3. keep your hips on the floor while you straighten your arms, lifting your chest up off the floor

4. bend your arms at the elbow to gently lower yourself back to the floor

5. repeat 5-8 times

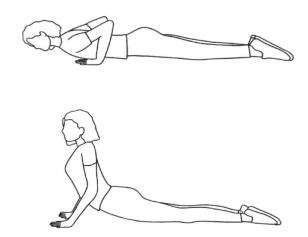

Wall Lean

Muscles targeted: oblique group, rotatores, intertransversarii, multifidus, and quadratus lumborum.

Step by step:

1. stand with your feet hip-width apart, with your healthy side facing the wall

2. bend the arm nearest to the wall at the elbow, creating a 90-degree angle

3. rest the length of your forearm against the wall, horizontal to the floor

4. lean towards the wall, shoulders first

5. rest the arm furthest from the wall on your hip, and gently push your torso towards the wall, creating a side curve of the spine

6. allow your hips to return to center

7. repeat 5-8 times

Aim to create a soft side curve to the torso, you don't want to force it into a sharp angle as this can cause damage by over concentrating the stretch in a single place. A good way to ensure that you are the correct distance away from the wall to start, is to use the length of your upper arm, once your elbow is bent, as a guide. Lift your arm to shoulder height and move sideways towards the wall until you can comfortably touch it with the length of your forearm. Then, you can lower your arm slightly as you lean into the stretch.

If you find it difficult to stand to perform this stretch it can be adapted to be completed laying on the floor. Lay on your side with your healthy side towards the floor, prop yourself up on your elbow to create a bend in the spine towards the ceiling. To increase the intensity of the stretch, you can move your arm closer to your hips.

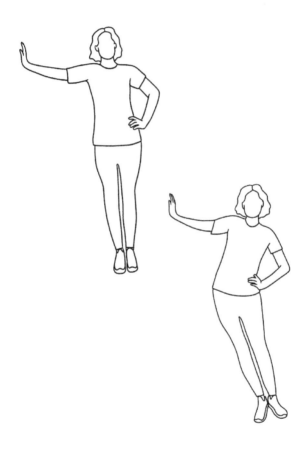

Chapter 12:

Five Bonus Stretches To Master

Deep Sumo Squat

Muscles targeted: erector spinae group, multifidus, latissimus dorsi, semitendinosus, semimembranosus, and gluteus group.

Step by step:

1. stand a few inches away from a wall, with your back to it and your feet a little further than shoulder-width apart

2. lean back onto the wall so that your back and shoulders rest against it

3. bend your knees and hips to allow you to slide your body down the wall

4. slide downwards until your bottom is below the height of your knees

5. hold this position for 30-60 seconds

This stretch can be difficult when you are beginning your stretching journey, you may want to move your feet further from the wall to reduce the intensity. Be sure to breathe steadily throughout, and control your movements so that they are slow and steady. The closer to the wall you position your feet, and the further down that you push your bottom, the deeper the stretch will be.

You may find it difficult to return to standing from this pose. If this happens, extend an arm out to the side, continuing to use the wall for support. Then, slowly slide yourself to the side and towards the floor. Once you are laying down, it will be much easier to un-curl your legs so that you can return to your feet.

After some practice, if you wish to challenge yourself, this stretch can be further adapted. When you reach the bottom of the position, you can clasp your hands and brace your elbow against your legs, an inch or two above your knees. Use your elbows to push out your knees, widening your stance.

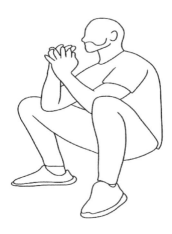

Seated Straddle

Muscles targeted: gastrocnemius, plantaris, soleus, semitendinosus, semimembranosus, erector spinae group, latissimus dorsi, posterior deltoid, quadratus lumborum, multifidus, gluteus group, quadriceps group, tibialis anterior, extensor digitorum longus, extensor hallucis longus, and intercostals.

Step by step:

1. sit on the floor with your legs straight out in front of you

2. move your feet apart as far as is comfortable to create a 'v' shape with your legs

3. place both palms on the floor in front of you, between your legs

4. breathe out and lean forward towards the floor

5. slide your hands across the floor, away from you, reaching forwards

6. hold this position for 30-60 seconds

For best results, slide your hands as far away from you as comfortably possible. Aim to keep your toes pointing to the ceiling, and avoid bending your knees. After some practice, you may find that you are able to move your feet further apart, or reach further forwards with your hands.

This stretch is a combination of the seated hamstring stretch and child's pose. If you are finding it too difficult, you can practice the two-component stretches individually and return to the seated straddle once you are more flexible.

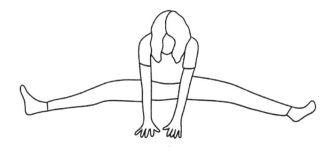

Iron Cross

Muscles targeted: oblique group, transverse abdominis, quadratus lumborum, erector spinae group, latissimus dorsi, and to a lesser extent, the pectoralis group, serratus anterior, and intercostals.

Step by step:

1. lay on your back, resting your arms out to the sides at shoulder level

2. lift your left leg, creating a 90-degree angle at your hip

3. keep your upper torso in place, breathe out and twist the lower torso to the right, until you can touch the floor with the inner side of your left foot

4. breathe in while you twist back to center, allowing your leg to follow the movement back into the air

5. lower your leg back to the floor

6. lift your right leg, creating a 90-degree angle at your hip

7. keep your upper torso in place, breathe out and twist the lower torso to the left, until you can touch the floor with the inner side of your right foot

8. breathe in while you twist back to center, allowing your leg to follow the movement back into the air

9. lower your leg back to the floor

10. repeat, alternating from side to side 5-8 times each way

This stretch uses the natural weight of your leg to increase the intensity of the stretch and is a more difficult variation of the laying T-twist. Aim to keep your back and shoulders against the floor as much as possible.

If you find it too difficult to complete the whole rotation without feeling strain in your abdomen, you can bend the leg at the knee, aiming to touch the inside edge of your knee to the floor instead of your foot.

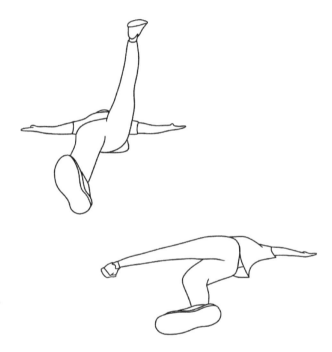

Quadruped Thoracic Rotation

Muscles targeted: rectus abdominis, erector spinae, pectoralis minor, lateral deltoid, latissimus dorsi, serratus anterior, levator scapulae, subscapularis, rhomboid, trapezius group, and subclavius.

Step by step:

1. kneel on the floor with your knees hip-width apart

2. lean forward, placing both palms on the floor, shoulder-width apart

3. keep your arms straight and your fingers spread to support your weight

4. raise your left hand out to the side of your torso

5. breathe in as you continue to raise your hand up, pointing your fingers towards the ceiling and rotating your torso to the left until both of your arms form a straight line through your shoulders

6. breathe out as you twist your torso back to the center and lower your arm.

7. tuck your left arm underneath your right arm, with the back of your hand towards the floor

8. continue twisting your torso, this time though to the right, sliding your arm along the floor until your left shoulder is touching the floor

9. twist your torso back to the center and place your palm back on the floor.

10. lift your right arm out to your side

11. breathe in as you twist your torso to the right, raising your arm into the air, with your fingers pointing towards the ceiling

12. breather out as you twist back to center

13. tuck your right arm underneath your left arm, with the back of your hand towards the floor

14. twist your torso to the left, sliding your right hand along the floor until your shoulder touches the floor too

15. twist back to the center and place your right palm back onto the floor

16. repeat, alternating sides 5-8 times in each direction

Aim to create all of the twisting action in your upper torso, the goal is to stretch the muscles surrounding your rib cage and thoracic spine. Avoid pushing your arm behind you to get your hand into the air. A good tip to help you prevent this is to look down the line of your arm as you twist your torso, this encourages your torso to follow the direction that your head and neck are turning. On the downwards movement, follow your arm underneath and out to the other side, as if your arm were a thread that you are using to thread the eye of a needle.

If you are finding the stretch too difficult you can adapt the movements to reduce the intensity. Instead of pointing your fingers up to the ceiling, or your hand being the first body part to thread underneath the other arm, bend your moving arm at the elbow and rest your fingers against your shoulder. In place of your free hand, use your elbow as the leading point, this reduces the pressure on the torso, and the hand that remains on the floor to support you. You may see some variations of this where the hand is placed at the back of the neck. I don't recommend doing this, as it can lead to a tendency to pull the torso around using the neck as a lever, which can cause damage.

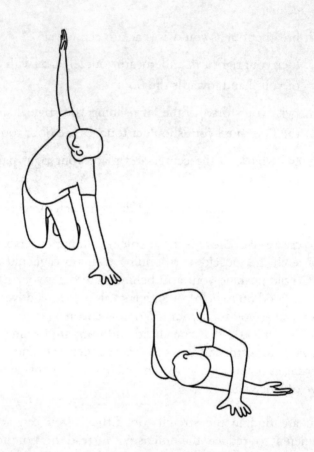

Seated Cross Shin

Muscles targeted: adductor group, vastus group, rectus femoris, pectineus, gluteus maximus, and to a lesser extent the digitorum group, hullucius group, tibialis anterior, and peroneus tertius.

Step by step:

1. sit on the floor with your legs in front of you

2. bend your legs at the knees and cross your legs at the shins

3. tuck your feet underneath your knees if possible

4. gently push your knees towards the floor

5. hold this position for 30-60 seconds

This pose is very relaxing and is a good finisher to an exercise routine. It can give you a moment to refresh your mind and rest before returning to the rest of your day. However, if you feel like you would prefer a bit more of a challenge, it can be adapted to increase the complexity. Once your legs are crossed at the shin, sit with your back tall and rest your hands on your knees with your palms facing upwards. This will stretch the muscles in your abdominal area, as well as open out your shoulders by externally rotating your arms. This is a great way to practice a healthy posture and is more challenging than you may think. Especially if you are guilty of sitting slumped in a chair, or spending a lot of time looking down at screens.

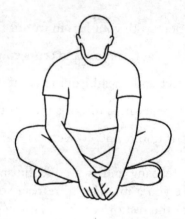

Chapter 13:

Extra Tools To Take Stretching

To The Next Level

Using A Foam Roller

The action of using a foam roller is a form of self-myofascial release (MFR). It is similar to giving yourself a deep tissue massage when you are experiencing soreness or tight muscles. The myofascial tissues are a network of fibrous tissue that surrounds all of your muscles and connects your joints, and bones. It also separates your muscles from each other and the other organs of your body, as well as holding your organs in place.

This tissue can become thickened and tighten around your muscles, reducing your ROM. The tightness caused can be a result of several things, most commonly you will experience it if you have been under active, or as a response to an injury. Myofascial tightness following an injury is your body's natural defense mechanism to protect the affected area by limiting the damage caused by extra movement. Sometimes though, this tightness can still remain after the injury has healed, and can be tricky to release. MFR aims to target these tightened fibers and encourage them to stretch back out so that your muscles can move more freely.

The results of using a foam roller to massage tightened areas are understudied, but early analysis indicates a number of benefits:

- reduced soreness following exercise

- increased flexibility and ROM

- reduce muscle pain

- increase relaxation

There is also some evidence that using a foam roller can temporarily reduce the appearance of cellulite, though isn't suitable as a permanent solution if this is an appearance issue that bothers you (Hildreth, 2021).

Some studies also show promising data that suggests MFR with a foam roller has positive effects in the management of Fibromyalgia symptoms (Ceca et al., 2017).

There are dozens of types of foam rollers available on the market today and they can be easily sourced online. Generally though, they will fall into one of the following categories:

- firm or dense

- medium firmness

- soft or low density

Additionally, foam rollers can be either smooth or textured, and some smaller varieties and roller balls are also available. Firm rollers provide the maximum pressure for the massage. If your pain is severe or chronic, using a foam roller may hurt at first. For this reason, it's better for beginners to start with a lower density roller until they get used to the process. Similarly, textured foam rollers will also provide maximum pressure, but are something that I recommend a novice avoid until they are more comfortable.

The primary use of foam rollers is as a tool that you can rest your body weight on top of, and then roll yourself on top of it, along the length of a muscle to coax the myofascial to release. They can also be used as stationary objects to encourage your body to increase the degree of a stretch; this is particularly useful for stretching the thoracic spine. A region that is typically difficult to exercise, due to the strength of the rib cage.

There are hundreds of beginners foam rolling videos online that will take you through a whole-body routine and how to ensure you have good form while doing so. I recommend spending some time watching a few to get to grips with it. However, there are also some basics that you need to know before you get started.

Always start your foam roller journey with slow and gentle movements; you may find yourself needing to adapt from tutorial videos, adjusting your body position to reduce the weight being placed onto the roller. Don't try to run before you can walk with this one, start small with 10-15 seconds of rolling in each location. Once you have achieved that and no longer experience discomfort you can increase your rolling time up to 30 seconds, and then 60 seconds at one time. As you become more practiced with the technique, you can also increase the pressure by introducing firmer rollers.

There are also some notes of caution that I must share with you, before you start. It is important that you never put pressure directly onto small joints with a foam roller. Avoid the knees, elbows, and any horizontal rolling across the spine to prevent causing damage to the ligaments and tendons surrounding the joints. That is not to say that you should avoid your back altogether, though; you can still practice using a foam roller in this area by ensuring the roller is vertically aligned to your spine, and you roll from left to right, as opposed to up and down.

For legs and arms, you can stay safe by applying the technique to your lower leg and then your thigh separately, and similarly, your upper arm and forearm separately, avoiding the joints in the middle.

As with any exercise, if the process causes, or increases existing pain, reduce the intensity, or stop. It is also important to stay hydrated, and you will want to keep a water bottle with you to sip throughout your routine.

Using a Lacrosse Ball

Lacrosse balls can be used to self- MFR in a very similar way to foam rollers. They are small, very dense, balls that do not compress when you apply pressure to them. There are some added benefits to making use of a lacrosse ball instead of, or as well as, a foam roller routine. Due to its significantly smaller size, you can use the ball to target areas of your muscles that are difficult to access with a roller. The lacrosse ball is especially good at MFR around the ends of muscles where they connect to the bones.

The lacrosse ball is placed beneath you, between your body and the floor, or trapped between your body and a wall, and then your body is rolled across the ball to massage the muscles and myofascial tissue. It is especially effective in treating your upper back and shoulders, when used with a wall for support. Another area that benefits greatly from the compact size of the lacrosse ball is the sole of your foot; by placing it on the floor and your foot on top of it, rolling your foot forwards and backward. The foot is a particularly difficult area to stretch for those who suffer from poor balance, so using a lacrosse ball while seated in a chair is a great alternative for those with plantar fasciitis.

Videos teaching the basics of MRF with a lacrosse ball are also abundant online, but there are some safety considerations to note before you begin. This technique is highly targeted to very small points of focus and can be more painful for beginners than foam rolling. If you experience severe pain, stop the exercise immediately. Avoid putting direct pressure on your knees, elbow, and spine. It is possible to work with the lacrosse ball on either side of your spine as opposed to directly on it, but I would recommend foam rolling for this area first. Always start small and build up from that foundation; begin with light pressure against your muscles for 5-10 seconds, then slowly increase your time by increments of 5 seconds at a time, up to around 60 seconds. Remember that hydration is key for good muscle health, and being dehydrated can increase the level of discomfort felt while practicing this technique.

Using Bands

Exercise bands - sometimes referred to as therapy or resistance bands - are elasticated bands that provide resistance for you to work against while stretching. It activates the muscles that are doing the work of the motion, helping you to build strength. Exercise bands can be just as effective as weight training, in building or maintaining muscle strength, which is an important accompaniment to gaining mobility through stretching. Using an exercise band is sometimes talked about as being like having a partner there with you to assist your stretching.

Exercise bands are highly recommended for seniors in place of a conventional weight routine, as it is gentler on your body and avoids placing excess weight on your limbs. It is also a perfect beginner's exercise tool, as it is inexpensive in comparison to other more traditional gym equipment. Exercise bands are a great way to add resistance to virtually any stretch position. Since they are small and versatile, I recommend packing one any time you go away for a few days so that you don't have to disrupt your stretching routine. These bands are often used in clinical settings or prescribed by physical therapists to rehabilitate patients following an injury, or surgery.

The many names used for exercise bands are partly due to their versatility of use, and partly due to the wide variety of types available. These bands are generally available in light, medium, or heavy resistance, and are color-coded, but they can vary from brand to brand, so experimenting a little at home to find the right fit for you may be necessary.

The simplest and often most inexpensive type of exercise band is a flat band. Flat bands are long flat strips of elastic material and are typically wider than any other type of band. A great benefit to these is that you can get them in almost any length so that you can use them when working full body positions. They are often cut into smaller pieces too, allowing you to exercise more fine movements, such as bending and stretching your fingers.

The next most common type of exercise band is the loop band. Loop bands are similar to flat bands, with their exception being that they are joined together at the ends to form a continuous loop of material. They are usually smaller and used mostly for limb mobilizations.

Resistance bands with handles, are things that probably take your mind back to the 1980s aerobics classes, and neon spandex suits, but they are still very relevant today and are a great alternative for anyone who would otherwise struggle to grip a flat or loop band. These bands are made up of a tube of elasticated material, terminated at either end with either a loop of non-stretchy material, or a solid grip handle. These types of bands are great at home substitute for the motions that are performed at a gym with a weight machine.

Less commonly used are leg or arm resistance bands. These exercise bands are a closed loop of the elasticated tube; some have a harder, more squash-resistant material inside them, so they can be used by either pulling or pushing on them. However, they are very specific in size and often limit the number of available motions or stretches that can be performed with them.

I already discussed one use for exercise bands in chapter 5: Lower Body Chair Exercises, when doing the calf stretch. I would also like to recommend an adaptation to the abdominal stretch found in chapter 8: Upper Body Floor Exercises, as follows: Before starting the step by step as listed for the abdominal stretch, place the middle of a flat or loop band, across the top of your shoulders, behind your neck. Take each end of the band in your hands and then perform the stretch as directed in chapter 8. The band will stretch as you straighten your arms, adding resistance to your back muscles which are doing the work of the stretch for you. This adaptation can help improve both standing and sitting posture by strengthening the back's extensor muscles. I especially recommend it if you spend a large amount of time sitting, which gives us a tendency to curl our bodies forwards.

Another adaptation to a stretch we have already covered that I would recommend is based on the calf stretch covered in chapter 7: Lower Body Wall Exercises. For this adaption, you do not need to use a wall, instead, sit with your knees hip-distance apart and your feet flat on the floor. Place the band under one foot, holding one end in each hand. Pull gently upon the band to assist you in recreating the toes to ceiling position of your ankle and hold for 30-60 seconds. This adaptation is a wonderful alternative for anyone who struggles to remain standing while performing the calf stretch or who have greatly reduced ankle ROM and need to start with a less intense option.

You can also reverse this process; instead of aiding your to stretch, you can use it to strengthen the muscles at the back of your leg responsible for lifting your heel from the floor at the beginning of your strides when walking. Sit in the position as described above, and pull on the exercise band to create tension on it. Then slowly push your toes to the floor, holding the band in place so that it resists your movement. Repeat this 5-8 times to strengthen your foot extension muscles. This is one of my favorite exercises, especially for anyone who has difficulty with their balance or who shuffles their feet when they walk. It improves your muscles' ability to create a confident heel lift from the floor on each stride and is an invaluable asset to your stretching routine if you struggle with getting forward momentum without becoming fatigued very quickly.

With these few examples, I hope that you can see where you too may be able to add a band into other parts of your stretching routine, that will be of the most benefit to your particular concerns or ailments.

Chapter 14:

Piecing It All Together

Now that you are armed with the functional knowledge of how to perform an effective stretching routine, let's take a look at how you can put it into practice. Stretching can be performed everyday, and some people who are confident with it can perform their stretches multiple times a day.

I recommend that you begin with just two to three times a week. Set yourself the goal of working up to being able to perform your routine every day. Your sessions do not need to belong in order to be effective. There is no need to try and squeeze stretches for every part of your body into one session, either. Targeted shorter sessions, working with one group of stretches at a time can actually be more beneficial.

Take some time to consider the condition of your own body; you know it better than anyone else. Consider where you feel the most restricted, and think about any areas where you experience pain that you would like to eliminate. These parts of your body should be the ones that you work on most often. Just 10 minutes a day, focusing on your own areas of weakness will be especially beneficial for you. If you have multiple issues that you want to address, you can target a different one in each session that you perform, and move on to the next problem area in the next session. The aim of this kind of narrow focus is to rotate between your areas of concern between each session that you perform.

How to Set a Routine

You can stretch at any time of the day and receive different benefits from doing so. But, starting any new activity can be challenging, so I recommend that you choose a time of day that you believe you can constantly stick to. While your favorite TV show is on, or while you wait for the coffee or tea to brew, is sometimes a good starting point, as you already have that time booked out in your daily routine, and you are simply adding a task to do alongside it. If you can't think of anywhere in the day that you can add your stretches into, consider purposefully clearing 10 minutes at the beginning or end of your day as an especially dedicated time for yourself. Performing your stretches consistently is key to the long-term benefits of stretching.

Planning your week ahead can be particularly useful in both dedicating the appropriate amount of time to your stretching, and in motivating you to check it off your list each day. I recommend using my free weekly planner for this reason.

Combining Stretches With Other Types of Exercise

While stretching is extremely beneficial for the health of your joints and muscles, combining a stretching routine with other types of workouts, has the potential to exponentially increase the benefits you can receive. If you are going to combine multiple types of workouts, I doubly recommend the use of my free weekly planner. Planning your week out in advance will allow you to see exactly what you need to do each day, in order to achieve your goals.

Stretching after a warm-up, but before a more intensive workout can reduce tension in the body and increase the effectiveness of your workout. If you wish to do this, it is important that you only choose dynamic stretches - these are the types where you gently move through a number of reps. The intention is that your pre-workout stretches will mimic the motions that your workout is going to cover, but in a slower, more controlled manner, like a signal to your muscles and joints that this is where they are going to be working as you continue your routine. Avoid static stretches - the types where you push into a position and hold for 30-60 seconds - as these can lead to injury when used right before intense exercise.

Conclusion

As our bodies age from the inside out, starting right at the cellular level, some decline in our health and flexibility is inevitable. But you don't have to settle for growing older and losing your ability to take part in activities you love. In this book you have seen how you can minimize the effects of aging, and reverse immobility problems caused through soft tissue injury or pain with a consistent, long term, stretching routine.

The benefits of adding regular stretching to your life include:

- reduced pain

- increased ROM

- improved flexibility

- improved posture

- increased energy

- increased relaxation

- improved mental focus

- reduced stress or depression

You are now armed with methods to create a stretching routine tailored to your own weakness and needs. From the correct set-up of your exercise space, where we covered the variety of mats that can create the right environment for you. Through step-by-step instructional guidance by type of stretch, giving you tips on achieving the correct form and staying safe while doing so. Then following the basics, I gave you more techniques and tools to take your fitness routine to the next level. All of this had the intention of helping you to create health goals that are bigger than you may have believed possible for you before.

You now understand some of the science behind common aches and pains, ailments that you have likely suffered from at some point too, and what you can do to address these difficulties in your life. I have shown you how to adapt stretches to both increase, or decrease their difficulty, so that you can build a stretching routine that suits your ability level and needs. I reminded you that, as always with any form of exercise, hydration is crucial. I can never overemphasize the importance of replacing the fluids that you lose during exercise. I covered with you any safety concerns wherever I feel they need to be a consideration, but always remember to consult with your primary care physician if you have any doubts. Stretching should be an enjoyable activity, and never create or worsen existing pain. Listen to your body, and don't be afraid to stop an exercise if something doesn't feel right, you can always adapt it to suit your needs in a less intensive manner.

An old Chinese proverb states that:

> The first step in a journey of a thousand miles, is the most important.

I believe that applies in many walks of life, but is particularly apt when it comes to health and exercise. It can seem daunting to be reminded that improvement takes time, and patience for consistency is key, but it helps to know that once you take that first step, the rest that follows will come more naturally because you already have momentum from creating the right mindset. Remember the reasons *why* you want to improve and not only *what* you want to improve; this is your motivator, without it you will have a tough time committing to getting better.

So, in closing, I encourage you to start setting goals today. Where do you want to be, and how do you want to feel, in the next four weeks? What about six months? Or even, a Year from now? There is no harm in thinking big, but stay organized if you really want to create that reality for yourself. Please visit my webpage now, to get your free copy of my weekly planner and start planning your new routine today. www.robertbalazs.com

"The best time to do it was yesterday, the second best time is now."

References

Avison, J. (2015). *Yoga: Fascia, Anatomy and Movement.* Handspring Publishing.

Baloh, R. W. (2018). *Sciatica and Chronic Pain: Past, Present and Future.* Springer International Publishing.

Bataineh, A. (2021, December 15). *Why we lose flexibility with age and what to do about it.* Span Health. https://www.span.health/blog/why-we-lose-flexibility-with-age-and-what-to-do-about-it

Besdine, R. W., & Alpert, W. (2020, January). *Changes in the body with aging-older People's Health Issues - MSD Manual Consumer Version.* MSD Manuals. https://www.msdmanuals.com/home/older-people%E2%80%99s-health-issues/the-aging-body/changes-in-the-body-with-aging

Bowen, V. (n.d.). *Maintaining flexibility with aging.* ARAPC. Retrieved April 26, 2022, from https://arapc.com/maintaining-flexibility-with-aging/

Brennan, D. (2021, June 15). *Myofascial release therapy: How does it improve tour health?* WebMD. https://www.webmd.com/pain-management/what-to-know-myofascial-release-therapy

Caring Healthcare. (2019, May 30). *Elderly stretching exercises benefits health in numerous ways.* Caring Healthcare. https://caringhealthcaresc.com/elderly-stretching-exercises-benefits-health-in-numerous-ways/

Ceca, D., Elvira, L., Guzman, J. F., & Pablos, A. (2017, July-August). Benefits of a self-myofascial release program on health-related quality of life in people with fibromyalgia: a randomized controlled trial. *The Journal of Sports Medicine and Physical Fitness, 57*(7-8), 993-1002. 10.23736/S0022-4707.17.07025-6. Epub 2017 Jan 31.

Chertoff, J. (2019, April 11). *Foam roller benefits, risks, and how to.* Healthline. https://www.healthline.com/health/foam-roller-benefits

Cordier, A. (2018, February 9). *5 reasons why warm up exercises are important-fit athletic - san diego best gym fit athletic — san diego best gym.* Fit Athletic. https://fitathletic.com/5-reasons-warm-exercises-important/

Creveling, M. (2018, January 23). *Ease sore muscles with these 5 lacrosse ball exercises.* Daily Burn. https://dailyburn.com/life/fitness/lacrosse-ball-exercises-sore-muscles/

Cronkleton, E. (2019, July 12). *Warmup exercises: 6 ways to get warmed up before a workout.* Healthline. https://www.healthline.com/health/fitness-exercise/warm-up-exercises#dynamic-warmup

Cronkleton, E. (2020, February 24). *Foam rolling: 8 magic Moves that'll relax all the tension in Your.* Healthline. https://www.healthline.com/health/fitness-exercise/foam-rolling-how-to#Be-careful-on-the-first-try

Department of Health, State Government of Victoria, Australia. (2018, August 22). *The dangers of sitting: why sitting is the new smoking.* Better Health Channel. https://www.betterhealth.vic.gov.au/health/healthyliving/the-dangers-of-sitting

Fossel, M. (2017). *The telomerase revolution: The enzyme that holds the key to human aging . . . and will soon lead to longer, healthier lives.* BenBella Books.

Fradkin, A. J., Zazryn, T. R., & Smoliga, J. M. (2010, January). Effects of warming-up on physical performance: a systematic review with meta-analysis. *Journal of Strength and Conditioning Research, 24*(1), 140-148. PubMed.gov. 10.1519/JSC.0b013e3181c643a0

Freutel, N. (2016, December 19). *Lacrosse Ball Massage: How to perform.* Healthline. https://www.healthline.com/health/fitness-exercise/lacrosse-ball-massage#Next-steps-

Freutel, N. (2019, October 15). *Stretching exercises for seniors: Improve mobility.* Healthline. https://www.healthline.com/health/senior-health/stretching-exercises#Chest-stretch-

Geriatric Medicine Journal. (2018, April 5). *Regular stretching is shown to improve muscles in elderly.* GM Journal. https://www.gmjournal.co.uk/regular-stretching-shown-to-improve-muscles-in-elderly

Golding, S. M., & Golding, L. A. (2003). *Fitness professionals' guide to musculoskeletal anatomy and human movement.* Healthy Learning.

Hansen, D., & Kennelly, S. (2017). *Plyometric Anatomy.* Human Kinetics.

Harvard Health Publishing: Harvard Medical School. (2019, May 23). *The dangers of sitting.* Harvard Health. https://www.health.harvard.edu/pain/the-dangers-of-sitting

Harvard Health Publishing: Harvard Medical School. (2022, March 14). *The importance of stretching.* Harvard Health. https://www.health.harvard.edu/staying-healthy/the-importance-of-stretching

Hildreth, D. (2021, December 22). *How to Get Rid of Cellulite on Thighs: Home Remedies and More.* Healthline. https://www.healthline.com/health/how-to-get-rid-of-cellulite-on-thighs

Holly, P. (2017, August 15). *9 reasons to use resistance bands for working out.* ProsourceFit. https://www.prosourcefit.com/blogs/news/9-reasons-to-use-resistance-bands-for-working-out

i'move Physical Therapy. (2019, October 14). *Exercise and aging: Why you need to keep moving - i'move.* i'move Physical Therapy. https://imovedaily.com/exercise-and-aging-why-you-need-to-keep-moving/

Indoor Cardio Pro. (2020, December 20). *13 Different Types of Foam Rollers.* IndoorCardioPro.com. https://indoorcardiopro.com/13-different-types-of-foam-rollers/

Kuschmider, R. (2021, August 17). *Tight muscles? Try a foam roller.* WebMD. https://www.webmd.com/fitness-exercise/features/foam-roller-workout

LagligAnabola.com. (2022, April 27). *What should I look for in a fitness exercise mat?* LagligAnabola.com. https://lagliganabola.com/en/what-should-i-look-for-in-a-fitness-exercise-mat/

Maund, E., Craig, D., Suekarran, S., Neilson, A. R., Wright, K., Brealey, S., Dennis, L., Goodchild, L., Hanchard, N., Rangan, A., Richardson, G., Robertson, J., & McDaid, C. (2012, March). Management of frozen shoulder: a systematic review and cost-effectiveness analysis. *Health Technology Assessment 2012, 16*(11), 1-243. 10.3310/hta16110

Mayfield, R. (2020, September). *Keeping hydrated for exercise | Health Information*. Bupa UK. https://www.bupa.co.uk/health-information/exercise-fitness/hydration-exercise

Mayo Clinic. (2021, October 6). *Aerobic exercise: How to warm up and cool down*. Mayo Clinic. https://www.mayoclinic.org/healthy-lifestyle/fitness/in-depth/exercise/art-20045517

Mayo Foundation for Medical Education and Research. (2020, August 1). *Frozen shoulder - Symptoms and causes*. Mayo Clinic. https://www.mayoclinic.org/diseases-conditions/frozen-shoulder/symptoms-causes/syc-20372684

Mayo Foundation for Medical Education and Research. (2020, August 1). *Sciatica - Symptoms and causes*. Mayo Clinic. https://www.mayoclinic.org/diseases-conditions/sciatica/symptoms-causes/syc-20377435

Nelson, A. G., & Kokkonen, J. (2014). *Stretching anatomy*. Human kinetics.

Page, P. (2012, February). Current Concepts in Muscle Stretching for Exercise and Rehabilitation. *Int J Sports Phys Ther., 7*(1), 109-119. https://www.ncbi.nlm.nih.gov/pmc/articles/PMC3273886/

Palastanga, N., & Soames, R. (2012). *Anatomy and human movement: Structure and function*. Churchill Livingstone.

Rubberbanditz, LLC. (2022). *Stretching with Bands*. Rubberbanditz. https://www.rubberbanditz.com/exercise/stretching-exercises/

Schermelleh, L. (2014, February 3). *Cell Division - Mitosis and Meiosis | Ask A Biologist.* Ask A Biologist |. https://askabiologist.asu.edu/cell-division

Swanson, A. (2019). *Science of Yoga: Understand the anatomy and physiology to perfect your practice.* DK Publishing. DOI 19 20 21 22 23 10 9 8 7 6 5 4 3 2 1 001–310296–Jan/19

Waehner, P. (2019, August 30). *Total body stretching routine with resistance bands.* Verywell Fit. https://www.verywellfit.com/total-body-stretch-with-resistance-bands-1231152

Walker, B. (2021, February 21). *What is stretching? How to stretch properly? When to stretch?* StretchCoach.com. https://stretchcoach.com/articles/how-to-stretch/

Wilcox, A. (2021, August 26). *Healthy aging: The increasing importance of movement as we age — Movement Physiotherapy.* Movement Physiotherapy. https://www.movementphysiotherapy.com.au/themovement/2021/8/26/healthy-ageing-the-increasing-importance-of-movement-as-we-age

Wood, R. (2008). *Isometric stretching for Athletes.* Topend Sports. https://www.topendsports.com/medicine/stretching-isometric.htm

9 781778 155573